Praise for *The Fric*

"*The Friction Factor* makes healthy living attainable with a simple system for creating sustainable changes through diet and exercise. In today's fast-paced society where time is invaluable, Tyler Martin provides a clear-cut process where even the busiest people can still make impactful changes to their overall health. As a healthcare professional, I value his holistic approach that promotes rewarding longevity versus the short-lived quick fix people often look for."

—Danielle DuPont, PT, DPT, RRS, NASM-CNC, physical therapist, Foothills Sports Medicine, Phoenix, Arizona

"*The Friction Factor* offers practical, relatable, and real-life guidance for casting your vision and building your healthiest life habits. It offers a solid overview for how to leverage behavioral science to reduce mindset friction and to find, start, and stick to your healthiest path forward!"

—Natalie Pickering, PhD, ACC, licensed psychologist and CEO, High Places Coaching and Consulting, Inc.

"*The Friction Factor* is an easy-to-read, educational guide to healthier living. The suggestions offered here for both exercise and nutrition seem to make practical sense for those with busy lifestyles and appear to be not very difficult to incorporate into day-to-day living, with the goal being to reduce the friction factor that many experience with more traditional exercise regimens and diet fads. This is also in alignment with a broad suggestion I use with patients—that is, to find the sticky factors that will not only allow initiation of exercise and diet modification but also promote continuation."

—Brent E. McEntire, MD, internal medicine and pediatric physician

"Maintaining an active lifestyle and building healthy exercise habits are key to strengthening muscles and bones, improving balance and brain health, and preventing health-related issues and long-term illness. *The Friction Factor* offers a simple, foolproof, systematic method for even the busiest of individuals to incorporate daily exercise and make it a sustainable life habit."

—Karen Brooks, PT, DPT, owner of Elite Physical Therapy & Fitness

"Tyler identifies and calls out a societal problem we are too busy to admit. He did his homework, consolidating over 110 sources to deliver his efficient and systematic way to overcome friction in diet and exercise. This book is designed to put you in the driver's seat to create better habits, a healthier lifestyle, and a better quality of life."

—Thomas Vollmar, DPT, PT, OCS, orthopedic physical therapist

"*The Friction Factor* is a great read for anyone who struggles to achieve and maintain their lifestyle goals. In addition to practical wellness tips, Tyler Martin weaves in the science of habit formation, which is essential for creating behavior changes that actually last."

—Kayla Payne, MS, health and wellness coach

"*The Friction Factor* breaks down the overall importance of nutrition and diet as it relates to health and fitness in a very basic, straightforward, and knowledgeable way. It offers a great way to understand macronutrients and micronutrients in order to build a core meal plan to manage a well-balanced diet."

—Mary Rodehaver, RD, MS, Manager, Profile Plan

The
Friction
Factor

The Friction Factor

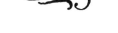

The Busy Person's Guide to Sustainable Diet and Exercise

TYLER MARTIN

Two Valleys Publishing

Two Valleys Publishing
www.twovalleyspublishing.com

Ordering Information
Quantity sales. Special discounts are available on quantity purchases by corporations, associations, and others. For details, contact the "Special Sales Department" at the address above.

Orders by US trade bookstores and wholesalers. Please contact BCH: (800) 431-1579 or visit www .bookch.com for details.

Printed in the United States of America

Cataloging-in-Publication data

Names: Martin, Tyler, author.
Title: The friction factor : the busy person's guide to sustainable diet and exercise / Tyler Martin.
Description: Includes index. | Louisville, KY: Two Valleys Publishing, 2023.
Identifiers: LCCN: 2022913943 | ISBN: 979-8-98640-20-4-8
Subjects: LCSH Exercise. | Weight loss. | Motivation (Psychology) | Self-actualization (Psychology) | BISAC
        HEALTH & FITNESS / Exercise / General | HEALTH & FITNESS / Diet & Nutrition / General
Classification: LCC RM222.2 .M37 2023| DDC 613.2/5--dc23

First Edition

28 27 26 25 24 23   1 2 3 4 5 6 7 8 9 10

Disclaimer: The diet, exercise, and lifestyle changes contained in this book are for educational purposes only and are not intended to be used in the treatment or prevention of disease or as a substitute for any exercise or diet plan prescribed by your physician or as an alternative to medical advice. All matters regarding your health require medical supervision. Please consult your physician or other health professional before beginning any diet or fitness program and about any condition that may require diagnosis or medical attention.

The exercise information contained in this book is to enhance and supplement but not to replace proper exercise training programs. Any form of exercise can present an inherent risk of injury. Before performing the exercises in this book, be sure that your equipment is well maintained, and do not take risks extending beyond your level of fitness, strength, flexibility, aptitude, endurance, or training. The author of this book advises readers to take complete responsibility for their safety and to be aware of their strength and endurance limits.

The dietary and nutritional information contained in this book is for educational purposes only and is not intended to replace a proper diet or nutrition program. Individuals seeking a personalized meal plan or grocery list should seek the services of a qualified nutrition professional. The author advises readers to take complete responsibility for all nutritional and dietary choices.

Every attempt has been made to present accurate and timely information. This field is constantly changing, which will account for many of the changes in references, resources, information, statistics, technology, approaches, or techniques that no doubt will occur by the time this book is purchased or read.

The author and publisher assume neither liability nor responsibility to any person or entity with respect to any direct or indirect loss or damage caused, or alleged to be caused, by the information contained herein, or for errors, omissions, inaccuracies, or any other inconsistency within these pages, or for unintentional slights against people or organizations.

Contents

Introduction   1

Part I: Winning the Psychological Game   9

Chapter 1: Motivation and Behavior Change   11

Chapter 2: Introduction to Building Exercise Habits   23

Chapter 3: Making Exercise Stick   35

Chapter 4: Timing Matters   55

Part II: Know Your Body and Set Your Goals   71

Chapter 5: Establishing Fitness Goals   73

Chapter 6: Managing Your Expectations   91

Chapter 7: Body-Composition Management   105

Part III: The Nuts and Bolts of Exercise   115

Chapter 8: Strength-Training Fundamentals   117

Chapter 9: Isolation Exercises, Cardio, and Exercise Selection   149

Chapter 10: Starting to Design Your Program   163

Chapter 11: Finalizing Your Workout Program   181

Part IV: The Nuts and Bolts of Diet and Nutrition

Part IV: The Nuts and Bolts of Diet and Nutrition   **197**

Chapter 12: Diet and Nutrition Basics   199

Chapter 13: Preparing for Meal Planning   215

Chapter 14: Building and Managing Your Meal Plan   235

Conclusion   257

Notes   259

Index   275

About the Author   283

Introduction

THIS BOOK WAS INSPIRED BY a powerful ideal: people can change their lives and pursue their happiness by taking the right actions. To fully embrace and benefit from this, I believe that to pursue and fully enjoy a good life requires a strong and healthy body. The purpose of any good life is not to tear down nor stand still—it's to build and create. My contribution to the ideal world filled with happy builders and creators is all the ideas that fill these pages.

How will this book help you? It will enable you to pursue a happier life by teaching you to conquer a massive barrier: physical fitness. Unfortunately, we're not born knowing how to get and stay fit. The plethora of different fitness approaches and advice can all seem confusing and contradictory. Without a clear and effective method of approach to physical fitness, most people are at an extreme disadvantage. *The Friction Factor* presents a happiness-oriented philosophy of fitness and gives a comprehensive roadmap for living that philosophy. If you embrace the system, you'll enable yourself to achieve more successes, give yourself more opportunities, and live more of the life you want.

I've learned a lot about living a healthy lifestyle since my days as a competitive athlete and coach. As a high school and college wrestler, I became acquainted with the arts of dieting, exercising, and maintaining a fit body at an early age. One of my primary jobs as an athlete was to stay in top physical shape so I could perform—and I had ample time and energy to do so back then. After retiring from athletics and venturing out into the workforce, I quickly realized that staying fit would become a substantial challenge. It was clear that as an average working person, I'd now have significantly less time and energy to devote to taking care of my body. Though I had many career and personal ambitions that required much of my time, the importance of physical fitness to my long-term happiness was also clear to me. I was convinced that to enjoy a long life of the highest quality possible, I must find a way to make the cultivation of fitness part of my everyday behavior. This created a significant challenge for me, and it's a challenge that you undoubtedly have too: how to fit diet and exercise into your busy life.

Initially, I didn't know how to solve this problem, but my time as an athlete gave me the first lead. It taught me that achieving long-term success at any skill requires developing the right habits. Training for wrestling showed me that developing habits requires repetition. To perform a difficult action with skill and precision against a tough opponent, you must have practiced it frequently and consistently. In the heat of competition, when I was exhausted and struggling for breath, what made it possible to continue taking the right actions was my habits. I relied on what I'd trained myself to do, the skills that I'd practiced thousands of times and didn't have to think about. When my habits failed to produce the desired effect, I didn't abandon them, instead I analyzed them to determine why the failure occurred. I adjusted and improved my methods but stayed committed to the process of habit building because when the pressure was on, my habits allowed me to prevail.

My time as a high school wrestling coach taught me that the importance of developing the right habits wasn't unique to me—it applies to everyone. Many of the athletes I coached had great success; the best claimed titles of state champion and All-American, and some went on to compete at the collegiate level. Most of them reached these heights in just four years of experience, surpassing others who'd been competing since they were toddlers. All these individuals succeeded because they learned to develop and sustain the right habits. This made clear to me that developing effective habits is a universal necessity for anyone seeking success in virtually any area. I resolved to apply this idea to solve the problem of fitting diet and exercise into a busy lifestyle.

As an athlete, I was motivated to do what was necessary to cultivate good habits because I loved to compete and win. To me, doing the work necessary to develop good habits was always worth the effort, and I could see the results of that hard work in my performance. This same dynamic exists when trying to improve your fitness by bringing diet and exercise into your life. You must understand exactly why fitness is important to you and have confidence that the actions you take will produce positive results. This theme reoccurs throughout the book. To build and maintain fitness habits requires a purpose that's meaningful to you and evidence you're making progress over time. The new approach to fitness you'll learn puts your life and values first, and it includes mechanisms for gauging your progress. The intent of this approach is to provide you with a philosophy and framework for fitness that fits into your busy life and can be followed for a lifetime. The principles, strategies, and tactics taught in this book are meant to be a reference tool that stand the test of time, a roadmap you can come back to when guidance and reassurance are needed.

In 2010, I began the serious endeavor of trying to select and implement the best fitness habits that would be effective and sustainable. After lots of trial and error, I finally discovered the two key ideas that made it possible to build optimal diet and exercise habits that fit into a busy life. After developing a system that worked for me, I spent five more years on how to present the system to other busy people—like you. It needed to be taught using simple principles and define what's necessary for long-term success.

I discovered the first principle by identifying what always kept me motivated to pursue fitness in the face of adversity. I asked myself, What has allowed me to keep dieting and exercising while building a successful marketing career, moving to different states, managing a small business, and writing a book? I realized I'm willing to put in the work that staying fit requires because I view fitness as a way to enhance my overall life. I believe that staying fit for a lifetime will make virtually every aspect of my life more enjoyable and of a higher quality. It will also make my life longer and provide me with more options for spending my time. This life-enhancing perspective of fitness is critical to staying consistently motivated to do the work that fitness requires.

The second key principle relates to how much time and energy you are willing to devote to pursuing physical fitness. For me, the biggest challenge of developing good diet and exercise habits was that everything I tried took too much time and effort. I just had too many other priorities to spend hours each day on fitness. While developing my system, I learned that I wasn't alone in this dilemma. More than 75 percent of Americans want to get more physically fit, but only 3 percent of them succeed at living a healthy lifestyle.[1] What are the main barriers preventing so many people from engaging in proper diet and exercise? Unsurprisingly, research shows that the most common reasons for not exercising or skipping planned workouts are lack of time and energy.[2] Likewise, the perceived complexity and time requirements for following a healthy diet are some of the most common reasons for not eating right. As evidence of this, one survey showed that 50 percent of Americans say that figuring out their income taxes is less complex than building a healthy meal plan.[3]

These widespread time and energy limitations are mostly process-related problems. Even though I was highly motivated, my time and energy were limited—like yours, most likely—so I needed to develop habits that maximized my limited bandwidth. To achieve this, I dissected my diet and exercising processes to discover where my time and energy were being used inefficiently. Throughout the book, the inefficient use of time and energy is referred to as *friction*. Friction stifles habit formation by unnecessarily increasing the amount of effort required to get the benefits of diet and exercise. When your process has too much friction, you lose motivation to continue. The key to sustaining fitness motivation is to eliminate as much friction as possible from diet and exercise. The comprehensive fitness system you're about to learn is built on this idea.

Chapter 1 of this book uses the first key principle—viewing fitness as an overall life enhancer—to help you map out the major benefits you hope to gain from improved fitness. It also explains the second key principle by demonstrating how friction can easily become a motivation killer. The subsequent chapters explain how to set appropriate fitness goals and build low-friction habits capable of helping you attain more of the life-enhancing outcomes that you want. Below is a brief overview of the key topics covered in these chapters:

Habit building—If you value what physical fitness can bring you, then you should establish the most efficient means of consistently achieving it. The key to doing so is turning fitness-promoting behaviors into *habits*. Habits economize your time and energy by automating behavior, reducing the amount of friction that pursuing fitness can cause in your life.

Physical requirements—To get healthier and more fit, the two most important habits to develop are effective dieting and exercising. Consistently exercise the major muscle groups via strength training, exercise your heart via cardio training, and eat a diet with adequate nutrition.

Diet and exercise strategy—Build a system of behaviors that has maximum impact but minimizes friction in your everyday life.

Exercise tactics—Use twenty-minute at-home daily workouts that include strength training and cardio to develop and keep lean muscle and cultivate a healthy cardiovascular system.

Diet tactics—Use a simple system of staple foods and core meals to minimize dieting friction, promote muscle development, and achieve healthy body-fat levels.

You know that learning to get and stay fit can be difficult. To make this easier, the book is organized to be a roadmap for acting. It walks you through the important ideas and steps to take chronologically so you can understand everything in context and as a complete system. In addition, the book provides many points where you can stop reading and take some action before continuing. For instance, you'll be asked to stop in chapter 1 to do some soul searching and consider how a lack of physical fitness might be impeding your happiness. Stopping to complete these exercises is crucial because it allows you to relate the abstract ideas to your concrete experiences. This allows you to build real understanding, set goals, and begin making strides toward better fitness as you read.

To make the content of this book as digestible as possible, it's broken into four distinct parts:

1. Winning the psychological game
2. Know your body and set your goals
3. The nuts and bolts of exercise
4. The nuts and bolts of diet and nutrition

The key topics of each part are organized into short sections to keep them digestible and easy to revisit for future reference. Each section uses as many example scenarios as possible to help demonstrate the real-world application of the ideas. Hopefully, when you read the examples, you'll think, "I've been in similar scenarios" or "I've had the same thoughts as the people in these illustrations." The intention for the book's presentation style is to demonstrate how practical *The Friction Factor*'s system is for busy people and how the system is different from most other solutions.

If you take nothing else from this book, remember these two axioms:

- To achieve and maintain physical fitness, be clear on how pursuing fitness will bring value to your life.
- The easiest way to consistently attain the benefits of fitness is to use the most efficient fitness methods.

These two ideas allowed me to solve my problem of how to fit diet and exercise into my busy lifestyle. As I began living by them, I was motivated to overcome the stress and pressures of life that derail so many people. In the face of twelve-hour workdays, client meetings, constant deadlines, running a small side business, writing, spending time with family, and the need for sleep, I still found a repeatable way to tend to my fitness. I became clear on what I wanted out of fitness and learned to eliminate friction from the process of pursuing it. At this point pursuing fitness became a lifelong habit for me, and by utilizing the same ideas and methods, it can become a habit for you too.

Unfortunately, understanding the big ideas isn't enough for you to achieve long-term success. If you think of pursuing fitness as a military battle, then the big ideas are the overall battle plan. Even with a great battle plan, soldiers can easily lose the fight if they don't know the right methods and tactics, such as how to choose the right weapons, attack, defend a position, or retreat. In the world of fitness, much of the friction that deters people from healthy dieting and exercising happens at the tactical level. How to fight lack of energy during workouts, how to quickly build a healthy meal when you don't have time for calorie counting, how to exercise while out of town on a business trip—these are all examples of tactical problems that can derail a great fitness strategy. Without a robust toolkit of fitness tactics, you will be overrun with such challenges and eventually lose motivation to pursue fitness.

How do you determine the right fitness tactics? The answer is that it often takes a lot of time and trial by error, which most busy people don't have the bandwidth for. Because of this, you might have tried other fitness systems in the past. If they worked well, then you wouldn't be reading this book. Why didn't they work? The main reason is that most popular diet and exercise systems don't make the issue of people's limited time and energy a strategic concern. Because of this, they don't scratch the surface of dealing with the friction people encounter at the tactical levels of diet and exercise. This book was written to solve that problem.

The Friction Factor gives you a fitness strategy—a battle plan—that's solely focused on addressing the primary reasons busy people fail at fitness: lack of time and energy. Based on this strategy, it teaches you the crucial tactical methods—a sort of soldier's field manual—for overcoming common sources of friction. These tips, tricks, hacks, and cheat codes are the secrets to eliminating friction from diet and exercise. Once you've mastered them, you'll be able to form lifelong fitness habits. What does that mean? It means that making the effort to pursue fitness becomes easier and part of your everyday life. It means that all the benefits you want out of fitness will come to you more consistently. Most importantly, it means that you can change your mindset and see the pursuit of fitness for what it truly is: an essential means of enhancing your life.

PART 1

Winning the Psychological Game

Part 1 is all about understanding how to establish lasting motivation and avoid the friction that stifles most people. It covers

- Fundamental strategies and tactics for building a repeatable exercise habit.
- The basic principles of where, when, and how often to exercise.
- Building new fitness habits so that the right behaviors feel virtually automatic—such as taking a shower or brushing your teeth.

By the end of this section, you'll have a unique new perspective on how to eliminate friction from the exercise process and set yourself up for long-term fitness success.

CHAPTER 1

Motivation and Behavior Change

THE BIGGEST CHALLENGE THAT MOST people face when trying to improve their physical fitness is a lack of motivation. You've probably experienced this in the past. Maybe you were excited about some new diet or workout program at first, but after a short time, the motivation faded. Lacking a sustained drive is a problem because to enjoy the benefits of healthy behaviors, you must be motivated to keep doing them. One of the main reasons people can't stay motivated is that they're not totally clear on what they're trying to achieve.

People's fitness goals are usually too vague. They'll make statements such as, "I want to get healthier," "I want to have more energy," or "I want to lose weight." These goals are great starting points, but they're not focused enough. To stay motivated long term, answer this important question: Why? Why do you want to get healthier? Why do you want more energy? Why do you want to lose weight? There must be specific reasons why you want these outcomes, and defining those reasons is required for staying motivated.

The following example demonstrates how defining *why* you want to get healthier can maintain your motivation. Bill is a sixty-two-year-old man who never put much stock in living a healthy lifestyle. His philosophy was "something's going to kill me one day regardless of whether I exercise and eat right, so I might as well eat, drink, and do what I want while I'm alive." For most of his life, Bill had no clear reason or goal to develop healthier habits. Everything changed after he narrowly survived his first heart attack. After that, it became clear to him that everything he cared about would be lost unless he adopted healthier behaviors. He'd lose opportunities to spend more time with family and friends and to pursue his hobbies and passions—all because his lifestyle was shortening his lifespan. Bill finally recognized the connection between health-promoting behaviors such as diet and exercise and attaining what he wanted out of life.

What can you learn from this example? Be completely clear on what you hope to gain from being fit and what's at stake if you aren't. You don't need to have a near-death experience to gain these insights, but you should put serious thought into what benefits the pursuit of fitness can bring into your life—and these benefits must be worth the effort in the long run.

If you already know exactly what you want out of pursuing better fitness, and you're 100 percent certain that these benefits will be motivational long-term, then you're in rare company. If you're like most people, you need some direction on selecting appropriate sources of motivation. Rather than guessing at what will motivate you, try examining the trouble spots in your life. You should identify the main ways that a lack of physical fitness might be causing you problems. The idea is to pinpoint how health- and fitness-related issues are making your life more difficult or unhappy. Identifying these trouble spots helps establish good sources of motivation because they usually indicate that something valuable is missing from your life. Finding sustainable motivation is much easier once you analyze and understand how *not* pursuing fitness is depriving you of life-enhancing benefits. While this approach may seem counterintuitive, it's an effective way to determine how pursuing fitness can make your life significantly better.

Let's look at some examples of how identifying the negative impacts of poor fitness can help uncover important benefits you're missing out on. Sandra, now in her forties, used to enjoy playing team sports. In high school, college, and her twenties, she played on many competitive and recreational volleyball and basketball teams. She especially enjoyed the camaraderie and friendships she developed through these activities and the confidence that came from honing and using her skills. Unfortunately, twenty years of office work and the demands of family life have caused her to become overweight, out of shape, and no longer fit enough to play team sports. Sandra's dissatisfaction with the lack of a cherished pastime—playing sports—and lack of confidence in her physical abilities have created a void in her life. She is depressed about the absence of the benefits she used to gain from sports and now has a dampened outlook for the future. She believes that as she gets older, her ability to get back to her cherished pastime is unlikely. In Sandra's case, poor physical fitness is depriving her of a highly valued type of social relationship and a source of pride and self-confidence.

Let's look at Jeffrey, a man in his late thirties who is seeking a romantic partner. He'd like to find someone nice and eventually settle down and start a family. Unfortunately, he is continually hindered in his romantic pursuits by his poor physical fitness. Most of the women that he's romantically interested in just don't find him physically attractive, and he feels very limited in his options. This is a major problem for Jeffrey because he values romantic love and companionship highly but is struggling to attain it due to his poor fitness. Just like with Sandra, the lack of fitness is depriving Jeffrey of results and outcomes that are important to him. Notice that in both examples, an especially unpleasant or unwanted type of experience—a trouble spot—helps point out when something important is missing from the person's life.

To help you identify the best sources of motivation, below is a list of eleven primary questions about your physical fitness and lifestyle. The questions were selected because they relate to some of the most common difficulties and dissatisfactions that people have in these areas. Consider each question and respond with either yes or no.

- Do you suffer from any lifestyle-related chronic medical conditions (e.g., diabetes, obesity, heart disease)?
- Do you lack energy on a regular basis?
- Are you uncomfortable with the appearance of your physique?
- Do you struggle with controlling your body weight?
- Do you feel physically weak?
- Does the state of your physical fitness ever cause you to feel unsafe or unhealthy?
- Do you experience a lack of self-confidence due to the state of your physical fitness?
- Does the state of your physical fitness degrade the quality of your romantic life?
- Does the state of your physical fitness cause you feelings of guilt or shame?
- Do you think your lifestyle choices will significantly reduce the length and or quality of your life?
- Do you think your fitness-related lifestyle choices are setting a bad example for your children, family, or other loved ones?

For each of the questions where you answered yes, answer the following two subquestions:

1. How has this limitation negatively impacted your life?
2. What would diminishing or totally removing this limitation enable you to do?

Remember that these eleven questions reflect just some of the most common problems and limitations that relate to health and fitness. If you experience other relevant sources of unhappiness or limitation, list them and ask yourself the same two subquestions about them.

Identify Your Motivational Sources

After completing the exercise, the next step is to use your responses to identify your most significant fitness-related trouble spots. To do this, pay special attention to how you answered each subquestion. The first subquestion asks you to explain how each difficulty or dissatisfaction negatively impacts your life. Doing so forces you to clearly identify some of your values you aren't currently living out—for Sandra it was friendships and self-confidence, for Jeffrey it was romantic love. The second subquestion asks you what the removal of each trouble spot would enable you to do. In other words, how would your life be better if the trouble spot were eliminated? This step is critical for establishing motivation because it helps you paint a mental picture of what your ideal life would look like. This is effective because, for most people, developing motivation for an outcome is much easier once they've visualized it. By considering your responses to this exercise, you'll be well on your way to visualizing the enhanced life that pursuing fitness can bring you.

Let's look at some examples of how examining your responses can help you paint a picture of a better life.

Example 1: Patricia

The primary question that stood out for Patricia was "Do you lack energy on a regular basis?" She answered yes.

- Subquestion 1: How has this limitation negatively impacted your life? Patricia's answer: "I often lack energy to play with my kids and help them with schoolwork when I return home from the office. My inability to do these activities has spurred frequent arguments with my spouse, which has negatively impacted our relationship."
- Subquestion 2: What would diminishing or totally removing this limitation enable you to do? Patricia's answer: "It would allow me to have the energy to play and interact with my children more regularly. It would also allow me to help more with their homework and remove a major catalyst for disagreements with my spouse."

In this example, Patricia believes that lack of physical energy is the result of her unhealthy lifestyle. This limitation makes it difficult for her to have the positive interactions she wants with family members. She identifies many ways that this occurs through her answer to the first subquestion. In response to the second subquestion, she says that having more energy would allow for better family interactions. For her, the motivating vision of an enhanced life is one where she has ample energy to put toward her family relationships.

Example 2: Reuben

The primary question that stood out for Reuben was "Do you struggle with controlling your body weight?" He answered yes.

- Subquestion 1: How has this limitation negatively impacted your life? Reuben's answer: "It has diminished my confidence in my appearance, which has made my demeanor more passive and reserved. I'm no longer comfortable with how my clothes fit, being photographed, or being in a bathing suit."

- Subquestion 2: What would diminishing or totally removing this limitation enable you to do? Reuben's answer: "I would be much more confident and wouldn't worry if people were judging my appearance. I would feel more comfortable in my own skin and engage in more social activities."

In this example Reuben identifies lack of self-confidence in his appearance as a significant limitation, which he believes is caused by being overweight. In response to the first subquestion, he cites several specific examples of how this limitation impacts him. In response to the second subquestion, he says that he'd be more confident and would engage in different behaviors if he could solve the problem. Based on his responses, Reuben's self-confidence is clearly impacted by his physique. For him, the motivating vision of a better life includes being much more confident in his physique.

Your Turn

Now use your responses to build a motivating vision of your future, one where improved physical fitness adds significant value to your life. First, identify the main ways in which a lack of physical fitness is negatively impacting your life. Then select the most powerful visions of how your life would be enhanced if those bad effects were removed. A word of caution as you form your life-enhancing vision: avoid making short-range fitness benefits a focal point of your vision. When the benefits of fitness are too short range, they won't be a sustainable source of motivation.

What is a short-range benefit? They are limited, time-bound advantages that come from improved fitness that generally have little or no lasting effect on your overall quality of life. For example, people often begin a fitness program so they can lose a few pounds and look good on their summer vacation.

The problem with making a short-term benefit (e.g., looking good for a few days on a special occasion) your primary source of motivation is that it has no staying power. Consider the real impact that something such as "making your goal weight" for vacation can really have on your life long term. Other than a few days of pride about your improved physique, there won't be a lasting effect for most people because the results are usually short lived.

The main problem with relying solely on point-in-time events—such as vacations, weddings, or pool parties—for motivation is that they are intermittent and infrequent. Where will your motivation come from when one of these special occasions isn't on the near horizon? When you take this approach, the answer is *nowhere*. When devoid of short-term motivation, most people revert to old—usually less healthy—behavior patterns until the next special event impels them to get fit. This ebb-and-flow type of motivation is one of the main reasons that people are constantly starting, stopping, and restarting fitness endeavors. If you've found yourself cycling between periods of exercising and then not exercising, dieting and then not dieting, feeling motivated and then defeated, you've been too focused on the short-term benefits of fitness.

How do you then avoid focusing on short-term fitness benefits? The trick is to identify the most significant ways you would benefit if the fitness-related trouble spots in your life were eliminated. As you do this, carefully consider which of these fitness benefits would continue to bring you long-term value. After putting some serious thought into this, select the top two or three benefits that you stand to gain from consistently pursuing fitness; choose the ones with the greatest capacity to increase your overall happiness. These benefits should be your primary sources of motivation. This crucial step forces you to reframe your ideas about fitness and begin thinking of it as a life-enhancing activity, not some chore or duty that you ought to do but dread.

Most people struggle to develop healthy behaviors because they don't see how doing so will really enhance their everyday life. In fact, many people view implementing healthier behaviors as extremely disruptive to their way of living. When you see that pursuing fitness will generate significant long-term benefits, finding and sustaining motivation gets easier, and you'll likely conclude that pursuing fitness might be worth the effort. In the next section, you'll learn about what's necessary to make pursuing fitness *always* worth the effort.

The Friction Factor

Once you know which long-term benefits will fuel your desire to pursue physical fitness, turn your attention to the challenge of implementing new behaviors. Most people implement new behaviors by forcing new activities into their routines without considering the potential negative impacts of those activities. In other words, they implement new behaviors without fully considering the compatibility of those behaviors with the rest of their life. For example, Heather gets motivated to exercise and lose weight as a New Year's resolution. She commits to hitting the gym for an hour per day after work. What she fails to consider is how this commitment will impact her other routines and activities.

After a few weeks, the long workouts and extra commuting time have made her evenings too hectic. She's staying up later to complete daily tasks, sleeping less, feeling more tired at work, and spending less time with her kids. After only a few weeks, Heather realizes the behaviors she's using to pursue her goal aren't sustainable, so she abandons her goal and quits going to the gym. This is an example of a crucial concept that was first mentioned in the introduction—*friction*. Friction occurs when the tactical behaviors you're using to achieve a goal cause too much disruption in your life to be sustainable. As friction increases, your ability to stay motivated decreases.

To make the pursuit of any goal sustainable, put special emphasis on selecting behaviors and tactics that minimize friction in your life. For example, using nicotine gum or patches is a lower friction tactic for quitting smoking than trying to quit cold turkey. Smokers who attempt to quit cold turkey usually will suffer withdrawal symptoms and be anxious and irritable, which can create a lot of friction. When the friction becomes too significant, they often relapse. In contrast, smokers using nicotine supplements to gradually wean themselves will generally experience less friction. They'll be much less anxious and irritable, so the new behavior that they've implemented—chewing nicotine gum—has less of a negative impact on their lives. Quitting cold turkey achieves the goal faster in theory, but using nicotine supplements is more likely to be effective because it causes less friction. In the same way, you can be more successful in your pursuit of fitness by being selective about the behaviors and tactics that you choose.

Let's look at how friction is a factor when it comes to pursuing fitness, even for people who are very fit. Daniel is a fitness enthusiast who loves exercising outdoors, but his employer just relocated him to a colder climate where he can no longer do this. This change of circumstance requires Daniel to change the type of workouts he does and the equipment he needs. To adjust to his new situation, he must consider how to continue pursuing his fitness goals without creating unnecessary friction. Here are a few examples of questions he might ask:

- Should I create a workout area in my house? Will this cause issues with my family by reducing our living space?
- Should I start exercising in a commercial gym? Do I have time to regularly commute to a gym? Can I afford to pay a gym membership long term?

Regardless of the solution he chooses, he should consider only new behaviors and tactics that don't cause significant friction in his life.

Where to Focus Your Effort: Diet and Exercise

Now that you understand the importance of choosing low-friction behaviors and tactics, the next question is, Where should you focus your efforts to improve physical fitness? The two crucial areas where new behaviors are required are diet and exercise. The right behaviors in these arenas will maximize your ability to control and improve your fitness. Most people fail to integrate diet and exercise into their lifestyle because the methods they select tend to generate massive amounts of friction. This is common because virtually none of the typically followed fitness programs are specifically designed to minimize disruption to everyday life (though some are better than others).

Why aren't common diet and exercise programs compatible with most people's lifestyle? The fundamental reason is that most don't put enough emphasis on the efficient use of time and energy. Here are a few common ways that popular fitness programs are disruptive to daily life:

- Many exercise programs and classes require
  - ☐ Traveling to a remote location
  - ☐ Working out for long sessions
  - ☐ Exercising at scheduled times (e.g., fitness classes or gyms with limited operational hours)
- Many diet programs require
  - ☐ Eating meals that require excessive preparation
  - ☐ Buying unusual foods that can't be found in most grocery stores
  - ☐ Adhering to a rigid meal plan, regardless of where you are and what foods you have access to

Common exercise programs are unsustainable for most people because they don't put an emphasis on economizing time and energy.

The result is the inefficient pursuit of fitness, which creates friction in many other areas of life. For instance, if your diet and exercise plan require a significant portion of your daily time and energy, you'll have less ability to pursue other interests such as personal relationships, family obligations, careers, or hobbies. When the pursuit of fitness becomes a barrier to a better life (rather than an enabler), it won't be sustainable. The key to creating sustainable diet and exercise habits is to select behaviors and tactics that maximize the use of your time and energy. In other words, select the methods that are most efficient.

Conclusion

At this point, you've identified how a lifestyle that includes diet and exercise can bring you significant life-enhancing benefits. You understand that the ongoing opportunity to gain those benefits is the best motivation to consistently pursue fitness and that you're not currently getting the benefits because you haven't formed the right habits. You also know that improving fitness means introducing new behaviors and that sustainable behaviors are those that minimize friction in daily life. Finally, you learned that most people fail to make diet and exercise sustainable behaviors because the methods they use aren't time or energy efficient. To overcome this challenge, you need a new approach to diet and exercise that focuses on minimizing friction and maximizing the use of your time and energy. The rest of this book presents a complete and systematic method for doing exactly that. With the foundation you've gained in this chapter, you're ready to begin the journey that will result in effective and efficient diet and exercise habits.

CHAPTER 2

∽⊃

Introduction to Building Exercise Habits

LEARNING TO EXERCISE CONSISTENTLY IS essential to improving physical fitness. Nearly everyone knows this, but training yourself to do it can be extremely difficult. Just consider that about 80 percent of Americans who start an exercise routine in January feel defeated and more likely to quit after six weeks.[1] Chances are that you've started and stopped an exercise routine at least once in your life. Why is keeping up a fitness regimen so difficult? The first reason was presented in the previous chapter: people tend to make exercise commitments that create too much friction in their lives. The other major reason is that people tend to set unrealistic short-term goals. They hold goals such as losing twenty pounds in a month or gaining ten pounds of muscle in a month. When they don't have the rapid success they hoped for, they usually lose motivation and stop exercising consistently.

The Need for Habit Development

When people attempt to exercise regularly, they often put too much emphasis on how much exercise they do and how quickly they can realize physical results. Exercise volume and improving your physique are important in the right context, but what value are they ultimately if the results can't be maintained long term? The truth is that attaining and *sustaining* positive results requires making regular exercise a repeatable behavior pattern. Initially, getting your body engaged in some type of regular exercise is more important than how long you work out or how fast you make progress. This means, for instance, that consistently doing five to ten minutes of jumping jacks is better than committing to an intense exercise class that's not sustainable. In the beginning, taking the emphasis off intensity and physical results allows you to focus on what's most important: the development of an exercise habit.

The word *habit* was mentioned a few times in the previous chapter, but let's give it a formal definition and explain the importance of the concept. A habit is a behavior that's been repeated so often that it requires little conscious effort to be initiated or performed. The steps for executing these behaviors are stored in the long-term memory and are often cued or triggered by some external event or situation. Some good examples of common habits are activities such as brushing your teeth in the morning, showering before work, or reading before bed.

The primary benefit of habits is that they make the execution of repetitive behaviors more time and energy efficient because they require minimal conscious effort. They make many of our daily routines and tasks seem automatic because we don't have to think through everything step by step. You should be aiming to create this dynamic for your exercise. When you turn exercise into a habit, you address the primary reasons that most people fail to exercise consistently: lack of time and energy. Once working out becomes habitual, it'll begin feeling automatic and will require less mental bandwidth to complete.

Daily Exercise

With all this in mind, you should ask, What's the most efficient way to make exercise a habit? The answer is to do short *daily* exercise sessions. The reason for this is simple: habits are formed through consistent repetition. The more frequently a behavior is performed, the easier it is to make into a habit. Note here that the *frequency* of a behavior is much more important to habit building than the total amount of time spent engaged in the behavior. This means you're generally more likely to build a habit through short daily workouts than from longer workouts done less frequently.

Consider the following example. Anne does short workouts every day for a week (for a total of seven workouts). Chris does three much longer workouts during the same week. Though Chris spends more total time exercising, Anne initiates exercise more frequently than Chris—seven times versus three times. This means that she exercised 133 percent more frequently than he did. Anne is on the faster path to forming a habit because repetition is what instills the cues and steps of a behavior into the long-term memory. As the act of exercising becomes more ingrained, it will begin to require less conscious effort to initiate and will begin to feel more like an automatic reflex. This is what you want. With frequent repetition, exercise will come to feel extremely familiar, something that requires little thought or effort to initiate and engage in. If you exercise less frequently, it will feel unfamiliar and require significant conscious effort to initiate. In other words, less exercise frequency creates more exercise friction.

Problems with Lower Frequency Exercise Plans

Most traditional programs advocate training for three- to four-days-per-week for forty-five- to ninety-minute sessions. When taking this approach, you generally have certain days scheduled for exercise and certain days scheduled for rest and recovery. Here's an example of what this type of regimen can look like:

Monday: ninety-minute strength training and cardio
Tuesday: off day
Wednesday: ninety-minute strength training and cardio
Thursday: off day
Friday: ninety-minute strength training and cardio
Saturday: off day
Sunday: off day

While programs such as this can deliver great physical results, they allow people too many opportunities to juggle workout days and off days. The main culprit is the longer exercise sessions, which require a significant amount of time and energy. When life gets busy, people don't always have the time and energy necessary for long workouts. When this happens, they tend to say, "I'll skip my workout today and make up for it on a more convenient day." They might even commit to doing a double exercise session to compensate for skipping. This creates a significant challenge for busy people because they struggle to consistently find any convenient time to exercise, let alone forty-five to ninety minutes. The main dilemma is that lack of time and energy is being used as the justification for skipping workouts, but busy people often lack both. This results in people constantly waiting for the "ideal days" to exercise, but they rarely come. This mindset leads to quitting exercise for two main reasons:

- If you're exercising infrequently, then you will experience more friction when you work out because it's not habitual behavior.
- If you're exercising infrequently, you won't see significant results, which will drive you to ask, Are the infrequent workouts I'm doing worth the effort? When the answer is no, people usually give up on trying to exercise.

What does it mean if you constantly struggle to fit the traditional three- to four-day-per-week workouts into your life? It means that traditional exercise systems aren't compatible with your lifestyle; you're trying to fit a square peg into a round hole (which doesn't work). The solution is to ask a different question, which is, What type of exercise system is compatible with my busy lifestyle? The answer is one that creates minimal friction and is the most conducive to forming an exercise habit—which short daily workouts do best. While there's no way to completely remove the temptation to skip, the daily approach eliminates the feature of most exercise programs that encourages consistent skipping: off days. Keeping daily workouts short also removes much of the friction inherent in longer workouts because they require far less time and energy to get through.

To further support the daily exercise approach, research indicates that people who exercise daily are more successful at staying physically fit. For instance, the National Weight Control Registry keeps records of Americans who've lost more than thirty pounds and kept the weight off for more than one year. The data shows that 90 percent of those individuals exercise daily.[2] While weight loss and maintenance aren't the only measures of success, they're strong indicators that someone is in control of his or her physical fitness. Contrast this with the overwhelming number of people who set exercise goals every January and abandon them by March. Those in the latter group usually fail to avoid friction and form habits because (among other reasons) most of them are following a traditional three- to four-day-per-week exercise program.

Other Benefits of Daily Exercise

In addition to being best for habit development, daily workouts have other unique benefits that make them preferable to systems with off days.

The list below highlights some of these benefits:

- *Better mood and stress management*—Daily exercise helps you feel calmer and more content in stressful situations by increasing the production of endorphins and neurotransmitters.[3] Production of these substances increases after a bout of exercise and can have a lasting effect on your mood during the day.[4]
- *Enhanced mental capacities*—Twenty minutes of daily physical activity makes the regions of your brain responsible for learning and retaining memories work more efficiently.[5]
- *Increased energy*—Exercise can have an immediate effect on how fatigued you feel. The energy produced by the body at the cellular level is dependent on your daily activity level—more movement means more energy production.[6]
- *Better sleep*—Exercise increases the amount of deep sleep you get.[7] In addition, the stress-reducing effects of exercise can make falling asleep easier.
- *Curbed hunger*—An exercise session produces ghrelin and peptide YY, which are hormones associated with hunger suppression. Some research has also indicated that the increased body heat caused by exercise may help with appetite suppression.[8]

While following a three- to four-day-per-week workout plan can improve your fitness, it won't provide all these great benefits in the same degree as a daily program. The first reason for this is that because traditional programs don't prescribe daily exercise, they obviously can't provide all these health benefits daily. The second reason is that because traditional programs increase the likelihood of skipping workouts often, they also reduce the number of opportunities to get the daily benefits. The best way to maximize the benefits of exercise is to make it a sustainable habit—which is achieved most easily through short daily workouts. The fact that consistent daily exercise happens to provide additional health benefits compared to other approaches is just a bonus.

What about Rest Days?

A common objection to daily workouts is that they cause overtraining (putting undue stress on the body and increasing the risk of injury).[9] Of course, your body needs recovery time after exercise—especially after strength training. The easy solution is to work different body parts on different days. This is the same approach taken by traditional strength-training programs. They prescribe three to four unique workouts throughout the week that each focus on different exercises that work different body parts. The daily-workout approach just spreads these different exercises across a seven-day period. This provides plenty of recovery time for the individual muscle groups being worked if the program is properly designed.

While the daily workout approach doesn't allow traditional recovery or off days, every day is essentially a rest day for the body parts not being worked. In part 3, you'll learn exactly how to build a daily exercise program that adequately works the entire body without causing overtraining. For now, just know that a daily workout plan can be safe and effective for most people if properly structured.

Are Short Workouts Enough?

Another common objection to short daily workouts is that they aren't substantial enough to significantly improve your physical fitness. This just isn't true. The right exercises done consistently in twenty-minute daily sessions can help you get fit—though some people need to gradually build up to twenty-minute workouts.

The notion of effective twenty-minute workouts is foreign to most people because they believe that pursuing fitness requires regularly spending hours in the gym. A main source of this misconception is the assumption that improving fitness requires training like a competitive athlete. Most people think that since athletes train for long hours and they are fit, getting fit must require a huge time commitment. What's commonly missed in this line of thinking is the reason that athletes train for long hours. Their goal is to develop special skills and abilities for competition, and lots of training is the best way to achieve this. Improved fitness is just a positive side effect of athletes pursuing their primary objective (skill enhancement). This means that people attempting to train like athletes are taking an indirect approach, which is inherently inefficient. The twenty-minute-daily-exercise approach makes improved fitness the primary objective and the efficient use of time and energy the guiding principle.

Another common reason for thinking that long workouts are necessary is the belief that exercise is all about burning calories. Most people want to lose excess body fat; they know that burning calories results in fat loss and that workouts burn calories. This leads them to believe that they'll burn fat faster if they exercise a lot. This is technically true, but most people accept the idea out of context. For the average person, frequent long workouts are unsustainable because they cause lots of friction in other areas of life. Attempting lengthy workouts won't ultimately help much with fat loss because they're hard to do consistently. Instead, research suggests that you'll be more successful at reducing body fat by combining regular exercise with a calorie restricted diet. While short daily workouts alone won't bring all your fitness goals to fruition, they will deliver significant cardiovascular and muscle-strengthening benefits.[10]

How Long Does Habit Building Take?

Once you recognize the power of making daily exercise a habit, you'll ask, Will working out eventually begin feeling easier and a part of my normal routine? The answer is that while the physical labor of exercise basically stays the same, habit formation reduces the amount of mental effort that exercise requires. This happens because habits create psychological efficiency. As was said earlier in the chapter, repeating the process of exercise over time ingrains every step of your workout into your long-term memory. The result of this is that progressively it starts taking less mental bandwidth for you to get through the steps of a workout. When you reach this point, exercising requires much less active thought because you've memorized the process, making it feel familiar and automatic.

After accepting that having an exercise habit makes pursuing fitness easier, you'll probably ask, How long does habit formation take? Recent studies have shown that it can take anywhere from two to eight months, but on average, new behavior starts feeling routine and automatic after about sixty-six days.[11] Note that habits are formed *gradually*, which means that exercise won't be extremely difficult for sixty-five days and then suddenly become effortless on the sixty-sixth day. Rather, each workout gets a little easier as the process becomes more familiar. Eventually, it comes to feel as normal and routine as brushing your teeth or taking a shower.

If developing an exercise habit is taking longer than expected, you've probably overcommitted. Even if you value the benefits of exercise, the amount you've committed to might be creating too much friction in your life. Forcing yourself to do something that's not compatible with the overarching lifestyle that you want isn't sustainable. If you find yourself in this situation with daily workouts, the best solution is to reduce your exercise commitment. Remember, when trying to form an exercise habit, working out *frequently* is much more important than getting the *ideal* amount of exercise. This means that if you can't handle twenty-minute workouts in the beginning, you can shorten them to fifteen, ten, or even five minutes. When the goal is habit building, exercising for just five minutes per day is better than committing to something that you can't sustain long term.

If you need to begin your daily exercise journey with workouts that are less than twenty minutes, remember that you can build up to twenty-minute sessions over time. In most cases you'll feel encouraged to gradually increase time spent exercising as you begin solidifying the daily habit and experiencing success. For example, Kimberly has been doing ten-minute daily workouts for two months. During this time, she lost some excess weight, got stronger, and became comfortable doing short workouts. At the end of this period she said, "Doing ten-minute workouts is now easy for me, and the results have improved my life. I'm now willing to increase the length of my workouts to get even more life-enhancing results." Moving forward, she decides to increase the length of her workouts by one minute per week until she builds up to the twenty-minute mark. She could also try jumping right into fifteen-minute workouts to see if that's sustainable for her. The point is that while you may need to start slower, your personal threshold for what's repeatable will probably increase over time.

Note that certain life circumstances can arise that reduce the amount of daily exercise that's feasible for you. Even the most consistent exercisers can find themselves in situations that might require temporarily reducing their exercise commitment. Say you've been exercising for twenty minutes daily for years, but you have a new baby or are trying to get up to speed at a demanding new job. In these scenarios, temporarily reducing to fifteen- or ten-minute daily workouts is better than ceasing exercise altogether. Once you get your other priorities under control, you can ramp back up to twenty minutes.

Though sometimes temporarily shortening workouts is appropriate, this is *not* the same thing as skipping workouts. Doing shorter exercise sessions still supports habit building—outright skipping does not. A good analogy for maintaining the habit of exercise during difficult times is fueling a campfire when you have no logs. If you've ever made a campfire and run low on logs, you know that keeping a few flames alive with sticks and leaves is better than letting the fire go out completely. Why? Because turning a small flame back into a large fire is much easier than trying to spark a new flame. Habits are like flames; building on a small habit is much easier than creating a new one. Doing *some* daily exercise when life gets hectic still helps keep the habit alive. This makes it much easier to build back up to twenty-minute workouts later when your time and energy bandwidth improve.

Conclusion

Short daily workouts are the most effective way for the average person to achieve long-term fitness success. This strategy helps you maximize the use of time and energy and is the best way to develop a sustainable exercise habit. Daily workouts also deliver many unique physiological and psychological benefits that other exercise strategies do not. The next chapter explores many of the common ways that implementing an exercise routine can create friction and presents tactics for avoiding them.

CHAPTER 3

Making Exercise Stick

CREATING AN EXERCISE HABIT IS the best solution to the fundamental problem of a lack of motivation to get fit. The standard approach to creating motivation is to somehow generate it purely through willpower. This is exactly what people do when they make drastic commitments such as hitting the gym for ninety minutes per day. They believe they can consistently force themselves to get motivated by means of sheer determination. The problem is that this doesn't work long term, which is why most busy people's pursuits of better fitness fall by the wayside quickly.

Motivation is not some mystical force; motivation is *the reason that someone has for acting or behaving a particular way.*[1] Being motivated to do something simply requires valuing that thing enough to devote the necessary time and energy. *Forcing* motivation through willpower isn't effective because it requires you to attribute more value to something than you truly believe it to have. In other words, forcing motivation requires you to "fake it," to pretend to want something more than you really do. If you do this, you end up burning time and energy on something that you care about less at the expense of outcomes and activities that you care about more. This is a major problem. As mentioned in the first chapter, forcing radical behavior changes that make it harder to live the way you want creates friction and isn't sustainable.

The truth is that increasing your motivation to exercise will come only with time and experience. The reason bodybuilders and athletes are willing to spend so much time training is because they've come to value exercise more and more over the course of time. They've personally experienced the benefits, and they have extreme confidence that their methods and tactics will be effective. Once you experience losing some body fat or gaining strength, you'll probably begin seeing more value in exercise. When this happens, the potential for your motivation to increase can rise. For anyone just getting started, this means that the amount of motivation available to you is initially limited. This is the reason why people not willing to exercise for twenty minutes per day are better off starting with fifteen-, ten-, or even five-minute workouts. The most effective motivation strategy is to be honest with yourself about what you're willing to do.

Focusing on creating an exercise habit is the best way to leverage your motivation because it allows you to maximize your use of time and energy. This approach recognizes that your motivational bandwidth is limited and puts the emphasis on efficiency. With exercise, the idea is to make the process of working out as easy as possible so you can make the most of the motivation you have.

Succeeding with this approach requires reducing or eliminating the parts of the exercise process that use time and energy inefficiently. In other words, find ways to remove friction from the process of exercising. Friction stifles habit formation because it increases the amount of effort required to achieve the benefits of pursuing fitness; it makes the motivational cost of exercising unnecessarily high. By eliminating friction from exercise, you lower the motivational cost and can make the most of your time and energy.

The largest sources of friction in the exercise process tend to come from the many secondary activities associated with working out. Most of them help make it possible to exercise, but they aren't exercise themselves. Throughout this book, they are referred to as *supportive tasks* because they relate to and support the activity of exercise. Here are some examples of common supportive tasks that often come with exercising:

- Planning out your workout routine
- Packing up your workout gear
- Driving to the gym
- Setting up exercise equipment
- Waiting for a turn on a piece of gym equipment

In most cases, the friction created by supportive tasks creates the resistance people feel toward exercise itself. This happens because supportive tasks can make the entire process of exercise more difficult to complete.

Some people feel apprehensive about the activity of exercise. The difference in this case is that any negative feelings toward working out are often offset by the immediate benefits exercise can provide. Instant benefits, such as gaining a sense of accomplishment, enhanced self-confidence, and increased energy, make resistance to exercise easier to bear. In contrast, the friction caused by supportive tasks is difficult to bear because they don't result in instantaneous benefits. In fact, supportive tasks are several steps removed from the actual activity that brings benefits (exercise). They seem to just add to the length of the whole process and increase the amount of time and energy required. Unfortunately, most people follow exercise systems that require many supportive tasks, which in turn create unnecessary friction. This friction quickly becomes a major deterrent to working out and ultimately drives them to give up.

A great example of a low-friction process with few supportive tasks is brushing your teeth. The steps of completing this process are as follows:

1. Walk into bathroom (supportive task).
2. Get out the toothbrush and toothpaste (supportive task).
3. Apply toothpaste to toothbrush (supportive task).
4. Brush your teeth (the primary activity).

Notice that the supportive tasks (steps one through three) are activities that require very little time and effort. By step four, you are engaging in the primary activity: brushing your teeth. While brushing your teeth isn't necessarily an enjoyable activity, most people understand its immense benefits, and the effort required is low. This type of dynamic is needed in the exercise process if you want a repeatable workout plan that can eventually become a habit. While doing daily exercise will never be as easy as brushing your teeth, removing the friction of supportive tasks is a game changer. It allows you to get the most out of your motivation and makes it easier to work out consistently.

The rest of this chapter examines common sources of exercise friction and suggests the best strategies for curbing and eliminating them.

Proximity to Exercise Location

A significant source of friction for most people trying to exercise is their proximity to a workout location. Traveling to a gym or fitness class adds substantially to the total amount of time that exercise requires, which is a major problem. For example, some people have a twenty-minute commute to the gym. That means a twenty-minute initial drive time, plus their total time spent at the gym, and then another twenty-minute commute back home or to work. In this example, time spent commuting adds forty minutes to the exercise process—before even considering other points of friction. For someone doing twenty minutes of daily exercise, even a five- to ten-minute trip to a gym extends the length of the exercise process by 50 to 100 percent. Someone with a twenty- or thirty-minute commute would require *at least* an hour per day for exercising. Those living in more rural areas or large cities with horrendous traffic must often bear even more significant travel times.

To better appreciate the friction that proximity creates, consider the impact it would have on a simple activity, such as brushing your teeth. Virtually everyone is willing to brush their teeth daily when the process requires only a few quick supportive tasks that take seconds. But what if brushing your teeth in your home were impossible? How much more difficult would it be to sustain the habit if every brushing required a twenty-minute drive to the dentist? How many more people do you think would skip brushing in this situation? While disgusting, it seems obvious that more people would skip the task more often. This example demonstrates how proximity can add an enormous amount of friction to even a simple process. It should now be clear why proximity is a serious impediment to a much more difficult activity like exercise.

The best way to eliminate the friction of traveling to a remote workout location is to exercise in your home. This allows you to significantly reduce the total length of the process and engage in the primary activity (exercise) much faster. If your supportive tasks take ten minutes and your workout takes twenty minutes, then your entire exercise process only requires thirty minutes per day. Common three- to four-day-per-week exercise plans usually require workouts that last forty-five to ninety minutes, not including the travel time to and from the gym. A twenty- to thirty-minute commute plus a forty-five- to ninety-minute workout means a much more significant time commitment is required. These larger time commitments are harder to fit into a busy schedule and ultimately make forming a long-term habit much more difficult.

Some people say that traveling to a commercial exercise facility is worth the time because it provides advantages that you can't get at home. Here are just a few of the commonly cited advantages:

- Allows access to special equipment
- Provides motivation of a group environment
- Eliminates the need to make space in your home for working out
- Avoids the need to buy expensive at-home equipment
- Offers access to professional instructors and coaches

While commercial gyms and fitness studios do offer unique benefits, they're not ideal for habit formation. In fact, most of the apparent benefits of exercising in an offsite facility are ultimately eclipsed by the friction that travel time creates. Fancy equipment, professional trainers, and the presence of fellow gym goers are great, but none of these solve the main problem: lack of time and energy. From an efficiency perspective, working out at home is undeniably one of the most effective ways of reducing friction in the exercise process.

Expense of Gyms and Home Equipment

People often say that purchasing home-gym equipment is too expensive and that paying commercial gym fees is ultimately cheaper, but is this true? To answer, we must first ask, How much does an average gym membership cost? According to the International Health, Racquet and Sportsclub Association, the average gym membership in the United States is $52.10 per month ($624 annually). If you live in a larger city, expect to pay even more. For instance, the average cost of a gym membership in New York (at the time of this writing) is $134.50 monthly ($1,614 annually).[2]

With a general idea of what gym memberships cost, we also need to know the average costs of working out at home. To do this, we must consider the types of exercises that you'd need to do at home. My system proposes doing weight-bearing strength exercises to work the major muscle groups and basic aerobic exercises to work the heart. While you can spend thousands on fancy equipment to accomplish this at home, doing so is totally unnecessary. You can do all the essential exercises with just a few pieces of basic equipment that are relatively inexpensive. In general, an effective home gym needs the following:

- A floor mat of some kind
- A set of adjustable free weights
- An adjustable weight bench
- A bench press or squat rack

Chapter 8 gets into more detail about all the exercise and equipment options, but the following sections provide the basic requirements. Note that you should hold off on selecting or purchasing any equipment until you've read all the chapters on exercise. Also note that chapter 8 provides some alternative body weight and resistance band options for those unable to purchase equipment.

Floor Mats

Good floor mats are at least four by six feet wide, which provides enough room for doing many types of exercises. Using them reduces impact on joints, protects flooring and your equipment from damage, and muffles the noise that's created by exercise.

Interlocking foam floor tiles are probably the most cost-effective option. You can buy enough to create a four by six surface for less than

$30 and can increase the size of the mat by purchasing additional tiles. The downside with these mats is that they're thinner than other types of mats, so they provide less cushioning.

Large nonslip mats are made of one flexible piece of material that can be rolled up and stored. They come in a variety of different sizes to meet most space requirements, and most cost less than $150. Note that these mats do tend to be more susceptible to the wear-and-tear of daily use than other options.

Wrestling or tumbling mats are extremely durable and provide lots of extra cushioning. You can generally purchase an appropriately sized mat like this for under $300.

Adjustable Free Weights

A basic set of free weights generally includes weight plates of various sizes, a barbell (weight bar), and a set of dumbbells. You can purchase a brand new 135-pound barbell set with a standard seventy-two-inch bar, two dumbbell handles, and a 120-pound set of weight plates for less than $150. A set like this generally comes with enough weights for the average person to get started. Ex-athletes and those who are naturally more athletic, powerful, or larger may need to consider purchasing a heavier set with more weights. If you need more weight, you can purchase a similar 300-pound weight set for less than $200. Also note that you can buy additional weights if needed.

Adjustable Weight Bench

An adjustable bench is a versatile piece of equipment that allows you to do many different types of exercises. They are relatively small and can be purchased for less than $150. Make sure that the bench you select can be put into a totally horizontal position, a ninety-degree sitting-up position, and a declined position.

Squat Rack

A squat rack is another piece of versatile equipment that will allow you to do a whole host of important exercises. You can find an adequate rack for less than $100. Make sure that the rack has safety catches—also called *spotters*—which allow for doing many barbell exercises safely without a workout partner.

Cost Comparison

Now that we've identified the basic equipment required for at-home workouts, we need to figure the average cost of this equipment. The list below shows the approximate prices of each type of equipment and the total cost for everything:

> Large nonslip mat: $150
> Weight set: $150
> Adjustable weight bench: $150
> Squat Rack: $100
> Total: $550

As you can see, the average cost of all this equipment ($550) is less than the average annual cost of a commercial gym membership ($697).

While purchasing home-gym equipment is generally cheaper than paying for a one-year gym membership, the reoccurring costs also need to be considered. Home-gym equipment is generally a one-time purchase versus gym memberships, which have an annual fee. With proper care, the workout gear you buy should last well over ten years—some may even last a lifetime. The cost of a gym membership keeps reoccurring and increasing for as long as you utilize the service. Table 3.1 shows the total cost of a gym membership over a ten-year period with conservative 3 percent annual price increases.

Table 3.1

Average Gym Costs over Ten Years

YEAR	MONTHLY COST	ANNUAL INCREASE (3%)	ANNUAL COST
1	$ 52.00	$—	$ 624.00
2	$ 53.56	$ 1.56	$ 642.72
3	$ 55.17	$ 1.61	$ 662.04
4	$ 56.83	$ 1.66	$ 681.96
5	$ 58.53	$ 1.70	$ 702.36
6	$ 60.29	$ 1.76	$ 723.48
7	$ 62.10	$ 1.81	$ 745.20
8	$ 63.96	$ 1.86	$ 767.52
9	$ 65.88	$ 1.92	$ 790.56
10	$ 67.86	$ 1.98	$ 814.32
		Total:	$7,154.16

As you can see, the ten-year cost of a gym membership is over seven thousand dollars, which is exponentially higher than the cost of home-gym equipment. In fact, you could spend much more on a home gym and still save versus spending money on a gym membership. It should now be clear that having your own workout equipment at home can be much less expensive than belonging to a commercial gym.

Making Space for a Home Gym

Another common concern people have about working out at home is that they don't have space for exercising or exercise equipment. One reason for this concern is that people aren't clear on what types of exercise to do or what sort of equipment they'll need. These questions will be answered later in the book. For now, just know that even people with limited living space can make room for a home gym by making the right considerations and getting creative. If making space will be a challenge for you, considering the following questions can help you determine the best solution:

- Is there an area in your home being used for overflow or storage of some kind? In many cases, these areas are portions of an unfinished basement, a bonus room above a garage, or a utility room. These types of spaces can often be reorganized to accommodate a small workout area.
- Is there a space in your home that can serve a dual purpose? Entire rooms are often dedicated to one specific task or type of activity that don't always require the whole space. In home offices, for example, people generally spend all their time in one small section of the room (e.g., sitting at a desk or table). The rest of the floor space is seldom utilized and could be converted into a gym area. Other good examples of these types of spaces are laundry rooms, spare bedrooms, and garages.
- Do you need to take stock of and throw away unnecessary belongings? Making room for a small home gym often requires dedicating only a few weekends to decluttering or rearranging a storage area. In many cases, the key is parting ways with items you no longer need that are taking up space.

If these questions haven't convinced you that making space in your home for exercise is possible, consider the following examples from my own life. They demonstrate how to create a viable home gym in the face of real space challenges.

When I first left home for college, I moved into a very small house with three other people. Knowing the importance of exercising at home, I bought some free-weight equipment at a yard sale and set it up in my ten-by-ten-square-foot bedroom. While this wasn't ideal, it was functional and allowed me to begin ingraining the habit of daily workouts into my lifestyle.

Throughout most of my twenties, my wife and I lived in multiple two-bedroom apartments as well as a small condo. In each of these living spaces we let one room serve as an office, gym, and storage area, so it had a triple purpose. Though quarters were tight, we could fit a mat, rack, bench, and set of free weights. This setup allowed us to get legitimate full-body exercise without leaving home.

My wife and I once bought a small house, which we renovated while living in it. The house was less than nine hundred square feet and very old, and it had no large closets for storage. Aside from the limited space, our renovations kept many of the rooms off limits, so there was virtually no room for a home gym. Our solution was to move our workout equipment out into the detached garage, which became our temporary home gym. Though we did have to add a space heater for the winter months, our solution was effective.

These real-life examples show how you can make a home gym solution work if you think differently about your living space. If you're not willing to put forth the effort to create a home gym, revisit your responses to the personal motivation exercise in chapter 1. Ask yourself, Is the relatively small amount of effort required to set up a home gym worth the benefits that a long-term exercise habit can bring to my life? For most people, the answer is yes. Remember, the extra friction that having to travel to an offsite gym location creates is a primary source of friction in the exercise process. Setting up a home gym is one of the most (if not the most) important steps you can take to increase your chances of making daily exercise a long-term habit.

The notable exception to the principle of working out at home is for those who live within a few steps of a commercial gym facility. This often applies to people living in apartment or condo buildings that have an on-site gym. These scenarios can be exceptions because the friction normally created by travel time is minimized when it takes only a few seconds to access the gym. If you live in a two-hundred-square-foot apartment but your building has a full gym, consider using it. Otherwise, use the recommendations provided in this section to pick a good space in your home to serve as your workout area.

Dependence on Partners and Groups

Many people prefer a fitness studio or commercial gym setting because they like to work out with a partner or group. Those who favor a non-solitary approach either get motivational value from the presence of others or need assistance with their exercises. Despite these benefits, the important questions to ask yourself are, Do groups or partners solve the main challenges of turning regular exercise into a habit? Do they reduce the amount of time and energy that exercise requires? Do they reduce friction in the exercise process? The answer is no.

Most people fail to exercise consistently due to a lack of time and energy. Groups and partners have virtually no positive effect on how efficiently you manage your time and energy levels. So while nonsolitary exercise might provide moral support, camaraderie, or the ability to do specialized exercises, it doesn't solve the main problem. On the contrary, nonsolitary workouts impose more rigidity on the process, which increases the amount of time and energy that exercising requires. Here are two significant ways in which reliance on partners and groups brings additional friction to workouts:

- *Schedule limitations*—Partners and groups inherently require compromising on when you can exercise because multiple people's schedules are involved.
- *Time pressure*—Most types of nonsolitary workouts are longer than individual workouts because they're not optimized

for time efficiency. This is especially true of working out with a partner because it generally entails sharing and taking turns with exercise equipment.

Note that the above limitations don't just apply to commercial gyms, they also apply to home gyms. You can't avoid the schedule and time pressures that come with groups and partners by hosting your workout sessions in your home gym instead. The only way to fully eliminate the friction that others bring into the exercise process is by working out alone. Learn to consistently motivate yourself and exercise in ways that don't involve other people. This frees you up to work out in the most efficient ways and at the most convenient times for you.

Other Common Sources of Friction

Unfortunately, working out by yourself and at home won't eliminate all the unnecessary friction from the exercise process. Many other significant sources of friction exist, such as

- Picking out and changing into workout attire and gear
- Planning your workout routine
- Setting up workout equipment

These aren't the only sources of friction, but they are some of the most common ones that you should be equipped to deal with.

In many cases, single supportive tasks don't create significant friction. Often, the combined friction caused by multiple supportive tasks is what deters people from exercising regularly. Also note that the cumulative friction of many supportive tasks is often further amplified by other pressures of a busy lifestyle. For example, tasks such as planning your workout or finding your exercise clothes might seem much easier on the weekend than during the workweek. Why? Because people are generally bearing more friction from work and homelife activities during the week. This cumulative friction can make it much more difficult to squeeze in a seemingly simple task such as finding your gym shorts and shoes. During the weekend or while on vacation, however, the cumulative friction that you encounter is usually less, which can make small supportive tasks seem like no big deal at the time. Don't be misled by how harmless supportive exercise tasks can seem on those rare days when you're taking a break from the daily grind. To build an exercise habit, you'll need to be able to deal with these tasks amid the many other sources of friction inherent in everyday life.

The following sections provide effective strategies for mitigating the friction that comes with the most common supportive exercise tasks. These sections also give you a more general idea of how to deal with other types of supportive tasks that aren't directly addressed in the book.

Finding Your Workout Gear

Selecting what you'll wear for your next workout seems like a relatively low-friction task, and it generally is when circumstances are ideal. Unfortunately, real-world circumstances are less than ideal more often than we typically realize. Ideally, you would open your closet and all the required exercise attire would be at your fingertips. The right T-shirt, shorts, socks, and shoes would all be immediately accessible; and it would take just a few seconds to change and begin exercising. For average people, the following scenario is more realistic: when they open their closet, they realize that some of their gear is wet in the washer, some is in the dirty clothes hamper, and they can find only one shoe. When this happens, what should take sixty seconds can turn into a fifteen-minute ordeal, which is a major deterrent when you're short on time and energy. For busy people, this type of friction is enough to prompt them to skip a workout for the day.

How do you prevent the task of finding your workout clothes from being a major source of friction? The answer is to put new processes in place to ensure that putting on your exercise clothes is frictionless when you're ready to exercise. To achieve this, gather your attire ahead of time so that no matter what, finding clothes isn't a hassle in the moment when you're ready to hit your home gym. This approach works because it lets you deal with any significant friction (such as selecting attire) in isolation from the primary task (exercising). For example, some people do need ten minutes to track down all their clothes, but they do this well in advance of their actual workout. Though there's still friction involved with the supportive task of finding their gear, finding gear is disconnected from the activity of exercising itself. The result is that the gathering of gear has already been handled when it's time to work out, so this won't be a friction point that can deter people from exercising.

To create the habit of finding exercise clothes ahead of workouts, add it to an already existing chore such as selecting your outfits for the workweek. This behavioral technique is called *anchoring*. Anchoring a new behavior means performing it in close succession to a well-established habit; think of it as adding a new step to an old habit. This helps form a mental association between the ingrained habit and the new behavior. It takes little effort to remember to perform the established habit, and performing it becomes the cue that triggers your new behavior. Here are a few ways you could anchor finding your exercise clothes to an established habit such as selecting your outfits for the workweek. If you iron and set out your work clothes for the coming day every evening, take a few extra minutes to also choose your exercise attire. If you prepare all your work outfits on the weekends, extend this chore to include gathering all your exercise clothes for the week.

You could also anchor finding your workout clothes to other daily habits. For instance, you might decide to set out your workout clothes every night after dinner or right after brushing your teeth before bed.

If you don't anchor finding your clothes to another habit, you should at least complete this task at the same time every day. Setting a reoccurring daily alarm on your smart phone can be a great reminder to get this done. If need be, liven up the activity by doing it along with something enjoyable, such as listening to music, an audiobook, or a podcast.

Regardless of how you develop the daily habit of finding your clothes ahead of workouts, doing so is helpful for reducing friction in the exercise process.

Planning Your Workout Routine

Planning your workout routine (i.e., deciding which exercises to do during each workout) is an extremely prevalent source of friction for most people. Like finding your clothes, it should *not* be done right at the beginning of an exercise session—which is the approach most people take. They walk into a gym and ask themselves, What exercises should I do today? To answer this question properly requires a significant amount of thinking and decision-making, which requires considerable time and energy. If it takes you ten to twenty minutes at the beginning of every workout to decide what to do, you're significantly lengthening the exercise process. In other words, you're adding friction. To give yourself the best chance of forming an exercise habit, the situation needs to be the exact opposite. When it's time to work out, you should have very little decision-making to do; you should be able to get into the act of exercising as quickly as possible.

People short on time and energy often resort to choosing what exercises to do haphazardly during their workout. You especially see this in large gyms with lots of equipment options. Selecting exercises at random is easy, but it fails to ensure that the right body parts are being worked from one exercise session to the next. The other problem with selecting exercises at random is the negative psychological effect that it has. When you create a workout haphazardly, you're implying that you don't know what action is required to achieve your goal. Eventually, this will lead you to question whether exercise is even worth doing—because you doubt that what you're doing will be effective. This doubt-ridden mindset can quickly spiral into a complete loss of motivation.

Another way that people try to deal with the friction of not knowing which exercises to do is to search the internet for instructions right before a workout. The problem with this approach is that while great information is available online, a person's long-range strategy will still lack continuity. Selecting instructional content haphazardly is the same as selecting individual exercises at random. The only difference is that you're arbitrarily selecting an article or video with workout instructions instead of actual exercises, such as push-ups or jumping jacks. Likewise, haphazardly selecting instructional content has the same psychological consequences as picking exercises at random. It still results in doubting the effectiveness of your approach to exercise, which inevitably erodes motivation.

How do you avoid the friction of deciding what to do during each exercise session while also ensuring that workouts are efficient and effective? The answer is advanced planning. To ensure that the right body parts are worked at the right times, do certain types of exercises on a regular basis. The good news is that anyone can achieve this by cycling through a small number of different exercises over the course of a few (usually three to four) days. This means that you need a single multiday plan that can be repeated indefinitely (with minor modifications over time). Part 3 will give you all the details needed to develop such a plan. For now, just note that the key to eliminating the friction of not knowing what exercises to do is having a single program that you follow repetitively. This is effective because once your initial plan is constructed, you don't need to make any decisions about what to do at the beginning of each workout.

Prepping Equipment

Another common supportive task that creates significant friction is setting up your workout equipment. Once you know what exercises to do, make sure that the associated equipment is properly situated for use. This often entails tasks such as unrolling workout mats, moving barbells or dumbbells, and portioning out the right amount of weight for each exercise. Completing all these tasks requires additional time and energy that can be a major deterrent to the act of working out itself.

Like other supportive tasks, equipment prep is a mandatory prerequisite that must be done before you can exercise. Though it can't be avoided, it can be dealt with in advance of and separate from the exercise session so that it doesn't deter you from deciding to work out. As with selecting workout clothes, it doesn't matter when you set up your equipment for the next workout, it just needs to be done in advance of and apart from the exercising itself. Again, this approach separates the two activities so they can be dealt with in isolation from one another. I personally prefer doing any preexercise equipment setup in the evenings so that everything is ready for my workout the next day.

An important part of making equipment setup easier is knowing exactly how much resistance to work with for each strength-training exercise. In other words, know exactly how much weight to put on each weight bar, machine, or dumbbell. People often spend a lot of time trying to remember how much weight they used for each exercise in previous workouts. This is a problem because our memories aren't as accurate as we think, and using the wrong amount of weight or resistance makes exercise less effective. The best way to recall the right amounts of resistance is to simply log your performance results from every workout. Doing this means always documenting how much weight was used, how many repetitions were done, and how many sets were completed for each exercise. Having this information documented allows you to simply consult your log to see exactly how much weight you'll need to prepare for your next workout. Chapter 11 will go into more detail on how to track and document your performance. For now just know that doing so is a great way to reduce friction.

Conclusion

After reading this chapter, hopefully you see that forcing yourself to be motivated to exercise daily is not feasible. The best way to make daily workouts a habit is to find ways of removing unnecessary friction from the exercise process. As you've learned, most of the unnecessary friction comes from the many supportive tasks associated with working out—not from exercise itself. In fact, the friction caused by supportive tasks is often what creates the anxieties and apprehensions that deter people from working out. When you learn to deal with supportive tasks more efficiently, you eliminate friction and make consistently exercising much easier.

To recap, here are the most commonly effective tactics you can employ to reduce the friction caused by supportive tasks:

- Work out at home instead of commuting to a gym.
- Exercise by yourself, not with partners or groups.
- Find and set out your exercise clothes ahead of workouts.
- Have a repeatable workout plan.
- Prepare your weights and equipment ahead of the exercise session.

CHAPTER 4

Timing Matters

THE PREVIOUS CHAPTER TAUGHT YOU how to remove friction from the exercise process by doing supportive tasks more efficiently. Another major source of friction that doesn't relate to supportive tasks is the time of day you work out. When you choose to exercise each day is extremely important to habit formation, so this entire chapter is dedicated to the topic. While some people have a more flexible schedule than others, the average person has only a few general times each day where exercising is possible:

- Midday—the time when most people stop for a lunch break
- Evenings after work
- Mornings before work

The following sections assess how effective these three time periods generally are for helping you establish an exercise habit. Even if you regularly have other opportunities to exercise during the day (besides those listed), the final recommendation will still apply to you.

The Lunch-Break Workout

The main problem with exercising during a lunch hour is that it usually requires commuting from work to your home gym. This creates a lot of friction because commuting takes additional time, and most people have limited time midday to try squeezing in a workout. In many cases, people's employers allow only an hour-long lunch break, which really makes exercising a challenge—especially if you commute. When you consider that you'll probably have to shower and maybe get something to eat, the lunch break workout starts to look impractical.

In addition to the challenges already mentioned, the lunch-break workout can also create a lot of psychological pressure. The stress of rushing to get back to work on time will become a daily occurrence—which will make the experience of exercising extremely unpleasant. In fact, being under significant time pressure might cause people to skip a workout altogether—especially if they're busy. A last-minute request from a boss or client or a fast-approaching deadline is all it takes to create enough friction to deter exercise that day.

The Evening Workout

The main challenge most people face when they attempt evening workouts is the lack of energy. If you've worked all day, you're going to be physically and mentally exhausted in the evenings. This is a problem because exercising will be one of the most (if not the most) physically and mentally demanding activities you'll do all day. Lacking energy makes it much harder to stay motivated and greatly increases the likelihood you'll skip workouts. This means that you'll probably exercise less frequently, which makes it extremely difficult to develop a habit. To combat low energy, some people will take caffeine or other supplements. This only compounds the problem by making it more difficult to fall asleep later that night. Those who take this approach will be even more tired the next day (due to lack of sleep) and even more likely to skip their next workout.

Another challenge with evening workouts is the increased likelihood of conflicting priorities—especially for those who don't live alone. After a long workday, nighttime is generally when people handle tasks such as household chores, family obligations, or errands. These might look like attending parent-teacher night, doing laundry, or paying bills. Additionally, the evenings are when many people deal with the unexpected personal issues that can arise during the day.

When you attempt exercising in the evenings, you put time for exercise into direct competition with the time needed for all these other priorities. In many cases, the chores, errands, and family obligations will take precedence and exercise will get skipped. Overall, it should be clear that fighting low energy and a high likelihood of competing priorities tends to make evenings a bad time for working out.

The Morning Workout

The primary challenge of the morning workout is that it usually requires waking up earlier. The thought of rising earlier is appalling to many people, but the advantages of morning workouts far outweigh the inconveniences of getting up sooner. One reason early workouts are ideal is that mornings are the time of day when distractions and competing priorities are usually at a minimum. The longer you've been awake, the more people and possibilities you'll encounter that can influence how you'll spend your time.

Here's what an ideal morning workout looks like for Brandon: he wakes up, hits his home gym for a twenty-minute workout, and then gets on with his normal morning routine—getting the kids to school and heading to work. In the morning, he hasn't yet run into any coworkers, so he doesn't have any new urgent work tasks. He also hasn't interacted with his wife or kids—they're still asleep, so no new at-home chores or tasks have been generated. In the morning, Brandon just has his goal to complete a short daily workout. While your ideal mornings might look different from Brandon's, the point is that these hours are generally more shielded from distractions and friction. This means that mornings offer most people the best possible opportunity to consistently complete workouts.

Even if your lifestyle is atypical—such as for those who work nights—you can still leverage this basic principle: get your exercise done shortly after waking. This means that if morning time for you is two in the afternoon, you should still exercise "early" in the day. Doing so allows you to work out *before* you have that flat tire or you get an unexpected dinner invite that throws off your plan. The further into each day you postpone exercise—regardless of when you wake—the greater the likelihood that you'll skip exercising.

Aside from being a less distracting time of day, our capacity to make good decisions is better in the mornings. As each day wears on, these capacities are depleted. Roy Baumeister, professor of psychology and author of *Willpower: Rediscovering the Greatest Human Strength* likens our ability to exercise willpower and self-control to a muscle; the more we use the muscle, the more tired it becomes. This is known as *decision fatigue*, which is the deteriorating quality of decisions made by an individual after a long session of decision-making. You can't avoid making decisions all day, but you can optimize decision-making by making the most important choices when you're fresh. Baumeister writes, "Most people have more energy in the morning, so important decisions should be made then, not at the end of a long, hard day."[1] This suggests that if you view exercise as important, then choosing to do it will be easier in the mornings before decision fatigue sets in.

Morning Workouts Promote Good Choices and Productivity

Another benefit of morning exercise is that it teaches a powerful time management principle: do the tasks with the greatest potential to enhance your life first. This idea was widely popularized by productivity author Brian Tracy in his bestselling book *Eat That Frog!* Tracy uses this old saying to teach the principle: *if the first thing you do each morning is to eat a live frog, you'll have the satisfaction of knowing that it's probably the worst thing you'll do all day.* The idea behind this analogy is that the tasks most likely to enhance our lives are difficult, and most people procrastinate on difficult tasks. But, if you do the difficult activities first thing each day, you'll feel a sense of accomplishment that makes life easier to deal with and you happier.[2] This is what most people experience when they begin each day with exercise; they feel a sense of accomplishment for taking action to enhance their life. This reoccurring self-esteem boost sets the tone for your whole day and encourages taking more steps to enhance your life. In this way, morning workouts can be the catalyst to enhancing the way you manage *all* your time and priorities.

Morning Workouts Enable Positive Mental Associations

The sense of satisfaction and accomplishment that people get from successfully acting to improve their life is significant. The ability to take successful action is a primary source of self-confidence and has a major influence on our happiness and conception of what's possible. Exercising in the morning gives you the best opportunity to consistently experience these benefits (compared to exercising at other times). If you choose the morning workout approach, you'll be more likely to start automatically associating exercise with many of these positive effects and good feelings:

- Confidence in your ability to deal with all the challenges of the day
- Pride in the initiative you're taking to improve your fitness
- A desire to become proactive in other areas of life

Reaching the stage of automatically associating exercise with these life enhancing outcomes makes it that much easier to do daily workouts. Rather than having psychological resistance and apprehension, you'll feel encouraged to engage in the activity. This is a far cry from the negative mental associations that most people form with exercise. Unfortunately, people tend to associate exercise with negative mental states such as anxiety, stress, guilt, or shame. Exercising in the mornings can be a huge help in changing your automatic emotional associations with exercise toward more positive mental reactions.

As you are hopefully now recognizing, the time of day that you work out can be a strong contributor to the amount of friction in your exercise process. By working out shortly after waking, you'll give yourself more opportunity to reduce friction and increase the likelihood of building a long-term habit.

How to Set Yourself Up for Morning Exercise

After exploring the many benefits of morning exercise, we must now explain how to make it part of your lifestyle. Before doing so, note that morning workouts are not absolutely necessary when developing an exercise habit. But the goal of this book is to present the best ways to eliminate friction from the process of getting fit, so we can't ignore that exercising in the morning is clearly a superior option—and the best option for most readers.

Tips for Saving Time and Getting to Bed Earlier

Most people are averse to morning exercise because it requires them to wake up earlier. This is a challenge because rising earlier can reduce the total amount of sleep that you get, and lack of sleep is already an issue for many people. In fact, 40 percent of Americans get less than the seven hours of sleep that the Centers for Disease Control and Prevention (CDC) recommends. Sleeping less than you already do so that you can wake earlier for a workout is not the right solution. Sleep deprivation can lead to many chronic health conditions such as heart attacks, heart disease, strokes, cancer, and diabetes. Lack of sleep also reduces mental sharpness and your ability to deal with stress.[3] The best way to get adequate sleep and take advantage of the benefits of morning workouts is going to bed earlier.

The main difficulty of going to sleep earlier is that it requires adjusting your nightly routine, which can be disruptive to your lifestyle. For example, going to bed earlier for the sake of morning exercise might require forgoing something else that you value, such as watching television or browsing social media. Most people view making such a change as a major sacrifice. To get past this resistance, reevaluate and consider what's truly in your long-term self-interest. This requires asking yourself the following questions:

- How much do I value forming an exercise habit?
- How does the value of the activities I do at night compare to the benefits that consistent exercise will bring me?
- Is it in my self-interest to spend less time on—or completely stop—some of the activities that are now part of my evening routine?
- Can any of the activities I normally do at night be done at another time to help me get to bed earlier?

After closely evaluating your evening routine, you'll probably find that it includes activities that you can forgo, do less of, or do at a different time. You might agree to watch one less episode of your favorite show or decide to start doing your social media browsing during lunch breaks. Sometimes, simple adjustments like these are all that's required to make bedding down earlier a possibility.

You should not stop doing activities that bring real benefits to your life. In many cases, activities such as watching a movie or television show, listening to music, or reading *can* be important to you. You don't necessarily have to give them up, but you should reassess how well they fit into your evening routine. Watching television and browsing the internet are activities people tend to do out of habit or as a pastime rather than as important activities they selected consciously. The point is that you can make it much easier to get to bed earlier by limiting or removing activities that don't add value to your evening routine.

If your evenings are full of important time-consuming tasks that must be done, try to do them more efficiently. Here are just a few ideas for speeding up common nightly tasks to help you get to bed earlier:

- Use a timer when doing nightly tasks. This prevents the mind from wandering, which makes getting chores done take longer.
- Minimize the need to spend time cooking by meal prepping or selecting foods that are easier to prepare.
- Use bank and personal finance apps to automate tasks such as paying bills and managing investments.
- Eliminate physical trips to stores whenever possible. Instead, have items delivered to your home (groceries, home goods, etc.).
- Limit the amount of time you spend doing tasks such as checking email or doing work-related projects in the evenings.

- Those with children of a certain age should teach them to engage in nightly chores and behaviors that help save time for the whole family. Enlist them to walk the dog, take out the trash, and do dishes and other various tasks.

These are just a few time-saving ideas. If you need more strategies or suggestions, there's a whole genre of literature and online content devoted to this topic. Find a good book, podcast, or YouTube channel that's devoted to lifehacks and saving time. Your overall goal should be to streamline your evening routine to make getting to bed earlier achievable. Doing this will allow you to get adequate sleep and make it much easier to rise earlier for daily workouts.

How Early Should I Get Up?

How much time do you need to free up in your evening routine? You need thirty minutes. If you can consistently get to bed thirty minutes earlier every night, then you can rise thirty minutes earlier and complete your daily workout. This approach allows you to get the same amount of sleep as you're used to, exercise, and go about your normal morning routine without disruption. People who fail to establish morning exercise routines are usually trying to get up much more than thirty minutes earlier, which causes a lot of friction. They must get up so much earlier because most morning routines require packing up gear, driving to a gym, checking in, planning a workout, and so on. These high-friction supportive tasks significantly lengthen the exercise process. Most people who work out in the morning must get up 90 to 120 minutes earlier, which generally isn't sustainable and makes habit building difficult.

Let's say people who had a previous wakeup time of 6:00 a.m. are now waking up at 5:30 a.m. Here's an example of what their new efficient morning looks like:

5:30 a.m.: Wake up and use restroom.

5:32 a.m.: Check body weight and other body metrics (more on this in later chapters).

5:35 a.m.: Put on workout attire and move to home-gym area.

5:40 a.m.: Begin twenty-minute morning workout.

6:00 a.m.: Begin normal morning routine.

As you can see, waking up and getting through a short daily workout in thirty minutes is possible, but making this behavior feel automatic takes time. (Remember that it normally takes about sixty-six days of repetition to form a habit.) A great way to help you adapt to new morning (and evening) routines is to write down all the steps on a piece of paper. Use these lists as a reference during these times to help guide you through the new processes until you get comfortable with them. Once you can easily get through the routines without referencing a list, you've probably begun to solidify new habits.

Tips for Getting Quality Sleep

Another tip to help you wake up earlier is to go to bed at the same time every night—especially on work nights. Doing so will bring regularity to your sleeping patterns and will ensure that you're rested enough to rise early and exercise. To regularly get to bed on time, establishing a step-by-step evening routine to follow is helpful. This bedtime routine should include all the essential tasks that must be done before you can go to sleep. In addition to completing all your critical tasks, a bedtime routine also acts as a cue to your body that it's time to wind down and prepare for sleep.[4] Your nightly procedure should generally include activities that help you relax, personal hygiene tasks, and tasks that help your mornings run smoothly. For many people, this includes tasks such as brushing their teeth, ironing clothes, or taking the dog out. Including preworkout tasks in your routine is also a best practice.

For instance, I always set up my exercise equipment as part of my nightly process. To remind you to begin your routine each night, try setting a reoccurring alarm on your smart phone to nudge you when it's time to get started. Here's an example of what a good bedtime routine could look like:

9:30 p.m.: Bedtime alarm goes off.

9:35 p.m.: Brush teeth and wash face.

9:40 p.m.: Set up weights and workout equipment for the next morning.

9:50 p.m.: Find workout clothes for next day.

10:00 p.m.: Lie down for the night.

Your routine might be different, but the main idea is to follow a set process at the same time every evening to ensure that you get to sleep on schedule.

A great feature to add to any bedtime routine is playing relaxing music, which helps you prepare for sleep. Generally, music without vocals is best for winding down because it's less jarring; it just plays in the background to set a calming mood. Music with lyrics tends to engage the listener and encourages singing along, which has less of a calming effect. Lots of great music in the ambient (nonlyrical) genre is good for relaxation. Slower paced classical music can also be great for relaxation. Try creating a nighttime playlist to use as a tool to help bring each day to a close.

Some activities to avoid right before bed are watching television, streaming online videos, surfing the web, listening to audiobooks or podcasts, or doing anything else that's mentally engaging. These activities can tempt you to continue watching or listening well past your planned bedtime.[5] This reduces the amount of sleep you're likely to get and makes it more difficult to rise on time for morning exercise. In addition to overstimulating your mind, most of these activities require looking at an electronic screen of some kind. The blue light put off by most of these gadget screens suppresses the body's production of melatonin. This is a problem because inadequate levels of melatonin can make it more difficult to fall asleep.[6]

Integrity of Your Sleeping Environment

Another important factor for getting adequate rest is the integrity of your sleeping environment. Anything in your bedroom or home (including other people) that disturbs your rest can sabotage your efforts to rise on time consistently for morning workouts, so try to identify and remove any sources of disturbance in your sleeping environment.

While many events can disrupt your sleep, the most common sources are mobile electronic devices such as smart phones, tablets, or watches. Many people sleep with these devices within arm's reach in case an emergency call or message comes through or because they serve as an alarm clock. Unfortunately, these gadgets also emit noises, flashes of light, and vibrations that can wake you up unnecessarily.

The straightforward solution to eliminating disturbances caused by mobile devices is to store them outside of the bedroom. The problem is that this eliminates the positives that they can provide (e.g., alarm clocks, getting emergency messages). For most people, the best option is to utilize the Do Not Disturb settings that are now standard on most of these devices. These special modes generally keep screens dark and mute all notifications and calls except from people on special contact lists that you can control. You can even program your devices to automatically switch to Do Not Disturb mode at specific times of day. For example, you might set your phone's Do Not Disturb feature to turn on every night at eight o'clock and turn off every morning at six. During this time frame, it would stay muted and dark unless a call came through from someone on your favorites contact list. As you can see, these features can be a massive help to ensure that mobile devices aren't waking you up at night.

Aside from mobile devices, many other environmental factors can make getting quality sleep difficult. Below is a list of some other common sources of sleep disruption and good remedies for dealing with each of them.

Room temperature—It can be very difficult to sleep if your bedroom temperature is too high. Make sure your room is in the ideal range for sleep—sixty-six to seventy degrees.[7] If necessary, get a small air conditioning unit for your bedroom to keep it cooler than the rest of your home.

Noise levels—General noise (from outside or inside your home) can be very disturbing. Block out such noise by running a fan or white-noise machine at night.

Pets—Allowing pets to sleep in bed with you is often a problem. The frequent movement of cats and dogs can cause you to sleep lightly and wake up often.[8] Train your animals to sleep elsewhere.

Other people—Family members coming in and out of the bedroom or otherwise making noise is extremely disruptive. If you live with or share a bed with others, make sure they respect your sleep schedule and environment.

Televisions—Having a television in the bedroom is often a big problem. They bring many of the same negative effects as mobile devices and can be detrimental to consistent sleeping patterns. Get televisions out of your bedroom.

Clocks—Old-fashioned alarm clocks cause many people anxiety, especially those who have trouble falling asleep. People tend to continuously check the time on these clocks and worry about how they haven't fallen asleep yet. If there's an alarm clock in your bedroom, face it away from your bed so that you're not tempted to incessantly check the time.

By assessing your individual situation and applying the advice provided in this section, you'll be able to get to bed earlier and get higher quality sleep. And getting better sleep makes establishing a morning exercise routine much easier.

Phasing in Morning Exercise

We've explored the many benefits of morning exercise, as well as many strategies and tactics for making it a habit. At this point, you might be wondering exactly when to begin getting up earlier. The answer is to implement morning workouts and new wake-up times at a pace that you're comfortable with. This means keeping your wake-up time proportional to the length of your daily workouts. If you've only built up the stamina for a five-minute daily workout, then you should get up early enough to exercise for five minutes. There's no need to start waking up thirty minutes earlier until you've developed the physical capacity for a full twenty-minute daily exercise session.

Let's look at an example of how someone should slowly integrate morning workouts into a daily routine. Michelle is just starting out with daily exercise. Initially, she can commit to only five-minute workouts. In this case, she only needs to wake up fifteen minutes earlier than normal every day. This provides her enough time to wake up and get through her workout without disrupting her normal morning routine. To slowly build her daily workouts up to twenty minutes, she decides to increase the length of her exercise sessions by one minute per week. As she does this, she likewise sets her morning alarm one minute earlier each week. After fifteen weeks, she is consistently rising thirty minutes earlier than before and working out for a full twenty minutes every day.

Conclusion

While morning workouts aren't mandatory for creating an exercise habit, hopefully you now see how much they increase the chances you'll form one. For most people, early mornings provide the only consistent window of distraction-free time when working out is possible. Exercising during other times (such as afternoons or evenings) invites friction and brings exercise into direct competition with other priorities. With morning workouts, you minimize the possibility of competing priorities and give yourself the best chance of creating a lasting habit. Additionally, starting each morning with exercise gives you a consistent source of accomplishment and sets a proactive tone for the rest of the day.

PART 2

Know Your Body and Set Your Goals

Part 2 is about gauging where you currently fall on the scale of bodily fitness, creating realistic targets for improvement, and maintaining your success. It covers the following concerns:

- What your basic exercise goals should be
- How to measure your current body composition and set future goals
- What's wrong with many popular myths about strength training and body composition
- How body fat and muscle mass can be controlled long term

By the end of this section, you'll have a great understanding of where you should be aiming when it comes to fitness and how to monitor and direct your continued progress over time.

CHAPTER 5

Establishing
Fitness Goals

SO FAR, WE'VE DISCUSSED why you should exercise, how long to exercise (twenty minutes daily), and when and where to do it (at home right after waking up). Now you're ready to begin setting some attainable fitness goals. Doing so requires learning some basic physiology and exercise science. Gaining this understanding will help you see how certain types of exercise can help you achieve your fitness goals. Building this knowledge base will also help you develop confidence in the new fitness habits that you'll be developing.

Basic Exercise Goals

Before you can set goals for your twenty-minute workouts, you should know what the two basic types of exercise are: *aerobic* and *anaerobic*. Despite the advice of many popular fitness programs, both sorts of exercise are required for achieving long-term fitness success. The following section provides an overview of the characteristics, benefits, and requirements of each.

What Is Aerobic Exercise?

When people are engaged in aerobic exercise (a.k.a. cardio exercise), their heart rate elevates and works overtime to deliver oxygen to their muscles. Anything that gets the heart pounding for a prolonged period is considered cardio. Some common examples of cardio workouts are running, swimming, dancing, and biking. These kinds of exercises make your heart healthier and more efficient at pumping blood through the body.[1] They also burn calories more efficiently than anaerobic exercise, which makes them a popular tool for weight loss within many exercise programs.

Why Is Aerobic Exercise Necessary?

Exercise is all about keeping your body strong so that you can navigate your life and achieve your goals. Building and maintaining a strong body requires exercising *all* your important muscles. Though the heart is an organ, you can also think of it as a muscle because it's composed of a significant amount of muscle tissue. The heart's muscular activity is crucial because the rest of your body—including other muscles—depend on it to deliver air and energy. To exercise the heart, regularly engage in some form of cardio exercise. Some programs proclaim that cardio is a waste of time, but this is a misleading statement. What most who promote this idea mean is that cardio isn't necessary for achieving certain types of goals, such as weight loss and building muscle. While this is true, note that cardio is also a requirement for *long-term general health*. In other words, cardio is necessary for staying alive longer, preventing disease, and maintaining a high quality of life. If living a long high-quality life is important to you, then skipping cardio is not an option.

How Much Cardio Is Necessary?

The American Heart Association currently recommends 150 minutes of moderate aerobic exercise or 75 minutes of high intensity aerobics per week.[2] Unless you're not healthy enough for general exercise or have been given different directions by a licensed professional, your basic cardio exercise goal should be to meet this recommended standard. If this sounds like a lot of cardio, don't fear! Subsequent chapters will teach you how to easily meet this requirement while only doing twenty minutes of exercise per day.

What Is Anaerobic Exercise?

Unlike cardio exercise, anaerobic exercise (a.k.a. strength training) does not primarily rely on breathing for energy. Instead, it draws energy from food-based fuel stored directly in your muscles and organs.[3] It does this because anaerobic activities require large amounts of energy at a very fast pace, and breathing isn't able to get the job done. Cardio requires slow-burning consistent energy, similar to the warmth a candlestick or campfire provides, so breathing works fine. Anaerobic activities such as strength training require large and explosive energy bursts, similar to the force a bomb or rocket creates, so they require a different kind of fuel.

Just like a rocket liftoff or bomb explosion, strength training uses up the available fuel quickly. As this happens, lactic acid begins to build up in the bloodstream. If you've ever experienced a burning sensation in your muscles while doing lots of push-ups or while hanging too long on playground monkey bars, then you've experienced a lactic acid buildup. The burn of lactic acid comes on very fast and quickly becomes unbearable. For this reason, most strength-training exercises can only be sustained for short periods—usually well under one minute. Some common examples of anaerobic or strength-training exercises are weightlifting, sprints, and push-ups.[4]

Why Is Anaerobic Exercise Necessary?

Strength training is necessary for long-term fitness because—aside from visually enhancing your physique—it enables you to enjoy a higher quality of life. The fact is that we all lose muscle mass as we age—this generally starts in our thirties. As this happens, we become weaker and less functional. By roughly age fifty, natural muscle breakdown often makes it difficult to do ordinary daily activities, which is detrimental to our quality of life.[5]

The best remedy for reversing muscle degeneration is building more muscle through strength training. This works because strength training stimulates muscle growth and causes you to become stronger.[6] When you're stronger and more fit, you're better able to move and engage with the world. This means more opportunities to gain or experience more of the outcomes you care about. In other words, strength training can allow you to have *more* of the life you want.

In addition to the benefits of enhanced muscularity, strength training also provides many people with emotional and psychological benefits. For instance, the experience of gaining physical strength, of being able to lift five pounds more than on a previous attempt, can be highly gratifying. This tends to raise your self-confidence and brings a unique sense of accomplishment.[7]

For some people, accepting that strength training is critical to long-term health can be difficult due to biases they hold. In many cases, people believe that activities such as weightlifting are base, brutish, or exclusively masculine pursuits—but they are mistaken. The fact is that people of all walks of life should work on developing strength and muscle mass because both are essential for living well long term.

How Much Strength Training Is Necessary?

Strength training is a primary tool for building and maintaining muscle so you can be fit and active and pursue your happiness for as long as possible. The American College of Sports Medicine says that people of all ages should practice strength training by exercising each major muscle group—arms, chest, back, shoulders, and legs—two to three times per week.[8]

Your basic strength training goal should be to meet this general standard. As with cardio exercise, the general strength training standard may sound like a lot, but again, don't fear! The subsequent chapters will explain how to meet the standard through short and efficient twenty-minute daily workouts.

Measuring Your Body Composition

Now that you know what your basic strength training and cardio goals should be, you can begin the process of setting your body-composition goals. Your *body composition* is the percentage of your total weight that comes from different substances such as muscle, fat, bone, connective tissue, and organs. The most important of these substances are body fat and muscle because they can be managed through diet and exercise. To effectively manage your body composition, select a goal for each of the following:

- Body-fat percentage
- Ideal body weight
- Muscle mass

The first step to setting these goals is to measure your current body composition to see where you are. To do this, take three key measurements: height, body weight, and body-fat percentage. Once you've taken these measurements, you'll be able to set realistic goals and will be well on your way to building a legitimate fitness plan.

Checking your height is the easiest of the three measurements to collect. If you don't already know your height, simply get a measuring tape, and use it to determine how tall you are.

The next measurement to take is body weight, which is also relatively easy. Obviously, the one thing you'll need to do this is a scale. If you don't own a scale already, go ahead and buy one; a scale is a critical tool for living a healthy lifestyle. While weighing yourself is a straightforward process that won't be explained step by step, here are a few general suggestions:

- Weigh yourself in the mornings when you have an empty stomach. Checking weight first thing each morning is also a great way to turn regular weigh-ins into a habit.
- Be sure to use the bathroom prior to stepping on the scale. This way food waste and liquid can't skew weight readings.
- Weigh yourself while completely naked. Clothes can skew weight readings and make them less accurate.

The third key measurement for assessing body composition is one that most people aren't familiar taking: body-fat percentage. The best way to measure body fat at home is using body-fat calipers, most of which are inexpensive and relatively easy to use. Calipers pinch skinfolds at multiple points on the body to gauge fat content. The measurements at these points are then used to calculate your total body-fat percentage. Calipers will come with detailed instructions on where and how to take the measurements. Note that the spots on your body for taking caliper readings are different for men and women and can vary between calipers. For example, many caliper systems require women to take three measurements: on the back of the arm (triceps), just above the hip bone, and on the thigh. Most systems have men take measurements in similar (but different) locations, such as on the pectoral area, abdomen, and thigh.

Be aware that body-fat calipers are less accurate for people with obesity (men with a body-fat percentage greater than 25 percent and women with a body-fat percentage above 32 percent). The reason for this is that obese people have a higher proportion of fat stored in internal body cavities that can't be reliably estimated with calipers. Despite being less accurate for people with obesity, these tools are still useful because they will reflect changes in body fat over time if used consistently. Plus, the readings will become more accurate as someone loses weight and falls out of the obese category.[9]

Nearly all calipers come with a calculator tool that use your age, sex, and skinfold measurements to calculate your total fat percentage, and all of them should be accurate enough for this exercise. You can find a variety of caliper options on e-commerce sites such as Amazon; they're also available at most health and fitness stores. Browse some of the available options, read some reviews, and then purchase a popular pair that are reasonably priced.

Note that most other methods of calculating body fat at home are *not* reliable. The most popular of these less effective options are digital body fat scales that can estimate fat percentage. These scales provide a rough estimate of your body fat by running a small electrical current up the leg. Sensors on the scale measure the amount of resistance that the current encounters as it comes back down the leg. This way of measuring fat is less accurate because it doesn't consider your height, stature, where you carry body fat, age, gender, or other factors that are important if you really want to know how much body fat you have.[10] One day these scales might be capable of taking more accurate measurements (which would be great), but they're not presently a good option.

Once you've calculated your fat percentage, use table 5.1 below to determine which category you fall into.

Table 5.1

Body-Fat Percentage Norms for Men and Women

Category	Women (%)	Men (%)
Essential fat only	10–13	2–5
Athletic	14–20	6–13
Fit	21–24	14–17
Acceptable	25–31	18–24
Obese	> 32	> 25

Source: "Percent Body Fat Norms for Men and Women," American Council on Exercise, accessed May 4, 2021, https://www.acefitness.org/education-and-resources /lifestyle/tools-calculators/percent-body-fat-calculator/.

After you take your three critical body-composition measurements, use them to estimate your current muscle mass. Due to the importance of muscle mass to quality of life, you should find out if your current muscle mass is low, adequate, or superior. The best way to calculate muscle mass at home is to use the fat-free mass index (FFMI). This index measures the amount of muscle in relation to a person's height. FFMI is similar to the more well-known body mass index (BMI), except that BMI is concerned with *total weight* in relation to height.[11]

You can manually calculate your FFMI using a series of formulas, but using readymade calculators available on the internet is easier and faster. The best solution is to use the FFMI calculator at frictionfactor fitness.com. From there, enter your height, weight, and body-fat percentage. Once this data is entered, the tool will automatically make the calculations. If you use another FFMI calculator, be aware that some may give you two different numbers: FFMI and adjusted FFMI.

If you encounter this, use adjusted FFMI to judge your muscularity because it factors your height into the calculation (regular FFMI does not). If you choose to calculate your FFMI manually, follow the steps described in table 5.2.

Table 5.2

Formulas for Manually Calculating FFMI

FORMULA NUMBER	MEASUREMENT	FORMULA
1	Lean body mass	Weight in pounds × (1 − (body fat percent ÷ 100))
2	FFMI	(Lean body mass ÷ 2.2) ÷ (height in inches × 0.0254)^2
3	Adjusted FFMI	FFMI + (6.1 × (1.8 − (height in inches) × 0.0254))

Source: Denise Nedea, "Fat Free Mass Index (FFMI) Calculator," MDApp, March 15, 2017, https://www.mdapp.co/fat-free-mass-index-ffmi-calculator-146/.

The first formula uses your weight in pounds and body-fat percentage to calculate your *lean body mass* (LBM)—which is the combined weight of a person's bones, muscle, connective tissue, and organs—with the total weight of body fat removed.[12] (If you use the metric system, you can easily make the weight conversion by multiplying your weight in kg by 2.205.) The second formula uses your LBM (in pounds) in relation to your height to calculate your FFMI. The third formula uses actual FFMI to determine your adjusted FFMI based on your height.

Tables 5.3 and 5.4 show two examples of how someone would use these formulas to calculate an adjusted FFMI:

Table 5.3
FFMI Calculation Example 1: Male

Height	5'11"
Weight	208 lb. (94.3 kg)
Body-fat percentage	30
Calculation 1	LBM: $208 \times (1 - (30 \div 100)) = 145.6$
Calculation 2	FFMI: $(145.6 \div 2.2) \div (71 \times 0.0254)^2 = 20.3$
Calculation 3	Adjusted FFMI: $20.3 + (6.1 \times (1.8 - 71 \times 0.0254)) = 20.3$

The FFMI (20.3) of the man in table 5.3 is identical to the adjusted FFMI because he is about average height (five feet eleven inches). Those who are shorter than five foot eleven (the baseline height used by the formula) will have an adjusted FFMI that is higher than their actual FFMI. Those who are taller than the baseline height will have an adjusted FFMI that is lower than their actual FFMI.

Table 5.4
FFMI Calculation Example 2: Female

Height	5'6"
Weight	159 lb. (72.1 kg)
Body-fat percentage	40
Calculation 1	LBM: $159 \times (1 - (40 \div 100)) = 95.4$
Calculation 2	FFMI: $(95.4 \div 2.2) \div (66 \times 0.0254)^2 = 15.4$
Calculation 3	Adjusted FFMI: $15.4 + (6.1 \times (1.8 - 66 \times 0.0254)) = 16.2$

Once you know your adjusted FFMI, compare it to table 5.5 or 5.6 below to determine which category of muscularity you fall into.

Table 5.5
FFMI Muscularity Scale for Men

FFMI	MUSCULATURE RATING
18	Slight build with low musculature
20	Average musculature
22	Distinctly muscular
> 22	Not normally achieved without weight training
25	The upper limit of musculature without pharmacological agents (e.g., anabolic steroids)

Sources: Christopher Eberley, "Hypertrophy Expectations," Kinesis Physical Therapy, January 23, 2014, http://exercisetoolkit.com/tag/fat-free-mass-index/; Roger Eston and Thomas Reilly, *Kinanthropometry and Exercise Physiology Laboratory Manual,* vol. 1, *Anthropometry* (New York: Routledge, 2009), 21.

Table 5.6
FFMI Muscularity Scale for Women

FFMI	MUSCULATURE RATING
13	Low musculature
15	Average musculature
17	Distinctly muscular
22	Not typically achieved without pharmacological agents (e.g., anabolic steroids)

Sources: Christopher Eberley, "Hypertrophy Expectations," Kinesis Physical Therapy, January 23, 2014, http://exercisetoolkit.com/tag/fat-free-mass-index/; Roger Eston and Thomas Reilly, *Kinanthropometry and Exercise Physiology Laboratory Manual,* vol. 1, *Anthropometry* (New York: Routledge, 2009), 21.

Setting Your Body-Composition Goals

After taking your current body-composition measurements, you're ready to start setting realistic body composition goals. The most important goals to set are

- A target body-fat percentage
- A target body weight
- A muscle development goal

The following three sections will show you how to set each of these goals.

Setting Your Target Body-Fat Percentage

For most women, the ideal body fat range will be somewhere within the fit (21–24 percent) and acceptable (25–31 percent) ranges. For most men, the ideal body fat range will be somewhere within the athletic (6–13 percent), fit (14–17 percent), and acceptable (18–24 percent) ranges (see table 5.1).[13] If you want a toned physique with visible abdominal muscles, then you'll need a body-fat percentage at the lower end of the athletic range (14–20 percent for women and 6–13 percent for men). Note that sustaining body-fat percentage above the acceptable range or below the essential-fat-only range can have severe negative impacts on your health. In some cases, these effects can even be life threatening. Also note that age is an important factor in determining what your body-fat percentage should be. Table 5.7 provides more detail on what the ideal ranges are based on age.

Once you know your ideal body fat range, you need to select a target body-fat percentage. If you aren't currently in the ideal range for your age, make your initial target to reach this category for your age and sex. If you're already in the ideal range and want to achieve

Table 5.7

Age-Based Body-Fat Guidelines

Age	Healthy body fat in women (%)	Healthy body fat in men (%)
20–39	21–32	8–19
40–59	23–33	11–21
60–79	24–35	13–24

Sources: Michael Woods, "Your Body-fat Percentage: What Does It Mean?" Winchester Hospital, October 26, 2016, https://www.winchesterhospital.org/health-library/article?id=41373; Dympna Gallagher, et al., "Healthy Percentage Body Fat Ranges: An Approach for Developing Guidelines Based on Body Mass Index," *American Journal of Clinical Nutrition* 72, no. 3 (September 2000): 699, https://doi.org/10.1093/ajcn/72.3.694.

a more muscular and toned physique, then set a target percentage in the athletic range—for best results—or at the low end of the fit range. Note here that achieving a visible six pack is *not* necessary for general health. For women, the lower limit for body fat is 10–13 percent—sustaining a fat percentage below this amount can have negative health consequences. For men, the lower healthy limit for sustained body fat is between 2 and 5 percent.[14]

If your body-fat percentage is above the acceptable range, your initial target should be to cut down to the acceptable category. Once you've achieved this, you can consider setting a new goal to reach the fit or athletic range if you choose. If your body-fat percentage is too low, you should work with a licensed medical professional to help you select an appropriate fat target. Based on your age and a variety of other factors, your doctor may recommend additional fat.

You now have all the information required to select your body fat target, so go ahead and set your goal. Once you've done so, congratulations will be in order because you'll be finished setting one of the three key body-composition goals.

Setting Your Target Body Weight

Once you've selected a target body-fat percentage, you need to calculate your target body weight. To do this, first calculate your lean body mass (LBM, see table 5.2). Once your LBM is determined, you can then use the following formula to calculate your target body weight:

Target weight = (LBM) ÷ (1 – target body fat percent as a decimal)

Tables 5.8 and 5.9 show some examples of the target body weight formula in use.[15]

Table 5.8
Target Body-Weight Calculation Example 1: Male

Height	5' 11"
Weight	208 lb
Body fat (percent)	30
Target body fat (percent)	22
LBM	145.6 lb
Target body weight calculation	(145.6 lb) ÷ (1 – 0.22) = 186.7 lb

The initial target weight for the man in the first example is 186.7 pounds, so he'd need to lose just over 21 pounds to hit his target. The target weight for the woman in the second example is 138.3 pounds, so she'd need to lose just over 20 pounds.

Table 5.9
Target Body-Weight Calculation Example 2: Female

Height	5' 6"
Weight	159 lb
Body fat (percent)	40
Target body fat (percent)	31
LBM	95.4 lb
Target body weight calculation	$(95.4 \text{ lb}) \div (1 - 0.31) = 138.3 \text{ lb}$

You now have all the necessary information to calculate your target body weight. If you haven't already done so, go ahead and calculate yours. Once this is complete, two of your three key body composition goals will be set.

Setting Your Muscle Development Goal

The final body-composition goal to set is your muscle development goal. Unlike your body-fat percentage and weight goals, your muscle mass goal should be directional rather than numeric. This doesn't mean you won't keep track of the amount of muscle you develop, it just means that a numeric target isn't necessary, so you don't have to set a specific goal, such as gaining five, ten, or twenty pounds of muscle. A directional goal indicates the general direction in which you want to make a change but doesn't specify the exact amount of change. For the average person seeking to get healthier and fitter, the two basic directional muscle goals to choose from are

1. Maintain current muscle mass while focusing on developing muscular strength.
2. Build more muscle mass while minimizing fat gain.

Setting a numeric goal for muscle development generally isn't advisable because everyone's capacity for building muscle is different. The speed at which you can build muscle and your overall capacity for doing so can vary depending on many factors, such as age, sex, or genetics. If you set a concrete goal, such as gaining fifteen pounds of muscle, and that goal is physiologically impossible for you, then you're setting yourself up for failure. In this situation, you'd begin losing confidence in your fitness program once it became evident that you weren't making progress. This could easily lead you to doubt the effectiveness of your program, which would be detrimental to developing healthy fitness habits.

The beauty of directional muscle development goals is that they are achievable for people of nearly all walks of life. By implementing the right behaviors, most people can maintain their muscle mass and develop some additional strength. They are also capable of building some additional muscle mass while minimizing fat gain if that's the goal they choose. Whichever goal you select, you'll see some degree of progress over time if you take the right actions consistently. Experiencing this progress will enforce the effectiveness of your program and increase the likelihood that you'll develop long-term habits.

Which directional goal should you choose, the first or second goal? To decide, take your current body-fat percentage into account. If your body-fat percentage is above the ideal range, focus on maintaining muscle and building strength (the first goal). Once you have reached your target weight and are happy with your body-fat percentage, you can then reassess your muscle development goal.

If you're happy with your current body-fat percentage and it's in a healthy range, then use your current FFMI to help you select an appropriate muscle goal. If your FFMI is in the low musculature range, consider making your goal to build more muscle mass while minimizing fat gain (the second goal). This is advisable because low musculature can easily become an impediment to a good quality of life—especially as you age. If you have an FFMI in the average range, you should also choose option two as your goal. In this situation, building additional muscle will help you hedge against muscle deterioration from aging and can deliver many other life-enhancing benefits (e.g., improved physique, additional strength, or more self-confidence). If you have an FFMI in the distinctly muscular range or above, use your own personal preference to decide on a muscle development goal. In this situation, you have plenty of muscle mass to sustain a high quality of life—if you take the right steps to maintain it. Most people who want to gain muscle beyond this point do so for aesthetic or physical performance reasons.

Now you can set your muscle development goal. Choose between option one and option two based on your situation. Once you've chosen a directional muscle mass goal, you will have completed the process of setting your three body-composition targets.

Conclusion

In this chapter, you learned about the two types of exercise that your twenty-minute workouts will need to include: cardio exercise and strength training exercise. You now understand why both types of exercise are necessary for good health, and you know what your basic exercise goals should be:

- Cardio goal: 150 minutes of moderate aerobic exercise per week—or 75 minutes of high intensity aerobic activity per week.
- Strength-training goal: practice strength training by appropriately exercising each major muscle group (arms, chest, back, shoulders, and legs) two to three times per week.

You've also learned how to take your three key body-composition measurements (height, body weight, and body-fat percentage) and use them to set your three body-composition goals:

- A target body-fat percentage
- A target body weight
- A muscle development goal

If you've completed all the instructions provided in this chapter, pat yourself on the back: you're one step closer to taking command of your physical fitness. If you haven't yet taken all your measurements and set your body composition goals, plan to do so as soon as possible. Establishing where you currently are and what your targets for change should be are crucial to consistently enjoying the life-enhancing benefits that improved fitness can bring. Also note that your body-composition goals will probably change over time, so plan to revise your goals as you become more fit.

CHAPTER 6

〜⌒つ

Managing Your Expectations

ONE OF THE MOST IMPORTANT keys to building and sustaining long-term fitness habits is learning to manage your expectations. A habit is useful only if it helps you get the benefits you're aiming for, so having a realistic perspective of what your fitness habits can deliver and how quickly they can do so is critical. Your fitness program should improve your physique and steer your development toward the goals you set in the previous chapter. If you think your program is failing to do this, then you'll eventually lose motivation to maintain your habits.

Unfortunately, people often believe that their efforts aren't paying off because they have unrealistic expectations of what's achievable. This chapter will provide you with the information needed to form realistic expectations about your body composition. The desired results don't always come as quickly as we'd like, but staying motivated is much easier when your results are aligned with reasonable expectations.

Your Total Goal Profile

The most important detail to recognize when setting expectations for fitness results is that your body-composition goals do not exist in isolation. Your target body-fat percentage, body weight, and muscle development goals all relate to and impact one another. This means that you need to think about these three goals as smaller components of a total goal profile. Thinking about your three targets as one goal profile makes it easier to grasp the dynamics of body composition and set more realistic expectations for results. Below is a list of some of the most common goal profiles people have:

- Lose significant body fat and maintain current muscle mass
- Lose moderate body fat and build moderate muscle mass
- Lose moderate body fat and maintain current muscle mass
- Maintain current body fat and build significant muscle mass
- Maintain current body fat and build moderate muscle mass
- Maintain current body fat and maintain current muscle mass
- Moderately increase body fat and build significant muscle mass
- Moderately increase body fat and build moderate muscle mass
- Moderately increase body fat and maintain current muscle mass

Body Fat and Muscle Mass 101

The key to understanding the relationships between your three body-composition goals is understanding the nature of muscle and fat. Remember, muscle and fat are the two tissues that you have the most ability to change through diet and exercise. Most people's goal profiles include body fat reduction *and* muscle development, so you should understand how these two processes can affect one another. If you don't, you'll never be able to set realistic expectations.

What Is Body Fat, and How Is It Controlled?

The best way to characterize body fat is to think of it as excess fuel that's being stored for later use. All the foods you eat are made up of substances called *macronutrients*; the three types are proteins, fats, and carbohydrates. Though each type of macronutrient is different, all of them contain *calories*, which are the basic units of energy that our bodies require for life. When you eat more calories than your body needs for energy, the excess calories are converted into body fat and stored for later use. This scenario is called *calorie surplus*. When you sustain a calorie surplus, your body-fat percentage and total body weight will increase.

Consistently eating fewer calories than your body needs for energy will reduce your body fat. This is called a *calorie deficit*. When this happens, your metabolism converts body fat into usable energy to get what it needs. In other words, if you don't eat enough calories, your body will "eat" its own body fat. When this happens, your body-fat percentage and total body weight will decrease. When you eat just enough calories to meet your body's energy needs, then your body-fat percentage and body weight will stay the same. This is called an *energy balance*.

Fat-Loss Expectations

If you're like many people, you may need to lose some weight by reducing your body fat. The first question to ask in this situation is, What should I do to reduce my body fat? As you've already learned, you need to create a calorie deficit, but this can be done multiple ways.

One popular method is to regularly do a lot of cardio exercise because more cardio can help you burn many more calories, which helps create a calorie deficit. Many people think the primary purpose of cardio is to burn calories for weight loss. Anyone who's ever visited a commercial gym in January has witnessed the pervasiveness of this belief. After the first of the year, thousands (if not millions) of people have weight-loss goals—which is why the lines to use treadmills and elliptical machines can become extremely long. They all believe that doing extra cardio is the best solution to burning calories. The problem with relying on cardio for weight loss is that it requires consistently exercising at a much higher volume than what's generally recommended.[1] The truth is that most people simply don't have the time or energy to spend many hours per week doing extra cardio. You might be able to do it for a few weeks or months, but the friction inherent in this approach quickly becomes unsustainable when life gets busy.

The most effective and efficient method for creating a calorie deficit for weight loss is to stick to a calorie-restricted diet. This method is preferred because it requires no additional time or energy. You simply decrease your calorie intake to an amount that's lower than your body's total daily energy needs. If you do this consistently, your body will use your excess fat as an alternative energy source. The result will be weight loss.

The second question to ask when it comes to setting fat-loss expectations is, How quickly should I expect to lose weight? The answer is that body weight can be lost very rapidly, but losing weight too quickly is generally considered unhealthy and unsafe. The maximum rate of weight loss that's widely considered safe is two pounds per week. Losing weight more rapidly than this can cause a significant amount of muscle loss as well as put you at risk for other health complications.[2] Rapid weight loss also increases the likelihood that you won't stick with your dieting plan long term.

If you need to reduce body fat, plan to do so by using a calorie-restricted diet and losing weight no faster than two pounds per week.

What Is Muscle Mass, and How Is It Controlled?

Muscle is a special type of tissue that can contract and expand, which allows you to move your body. When you put enough stress on muscles during strength training, they are exhausted of energy and structurally damaged. Your body then uses protein that you've eaten to repair the damaged tissue, which results in muscle growth.[3] To develop muscle mass, you must do adequate strength training and have an adequate protein-rich diet.

Muscle–Building Expectations

Recall from the previous chapter that your muscle development goal should be one of the following:

1. Maintain current muscle mass while focusing on developing muscular strength.
2. Build more muscle mass while minimizing fat gain.

People who choose option one will be trying to either lose weight or maintain their current body weight. This means that they will be dieting to achieve either a calorie deficit or an energy balance. Under these conditions, developing muscle mass is difficult because when your body is short on energy, it doesn't just rely on your excess fat. It can also cannibalize some of your muscle mass to get the fuel that it needs. In fact, it's estimated that about 25 percent of the weight that people lose comes from muscle loss rather than fat loss.[4]

As you now know, losing muscle mass is not good. You also know that being overweight is not good either. There's an obvious dilemma: the process of weight loss conflicts with the process of maintaining and building muscle. Luckily a reliable solution exists. You can prevent muscle loss during the fat-loss process by consistently doing strength training and eating a nutritious protein-rich diet. Some studies have shown that increasing muscle while in a calorie deficit is possible, but achieving this is not a certainty and you shouldn't generally expect such results.[5] If your initial goal profile includes fat loss, you should focus on eating right and not losing strength during the process. If you happen to build some muscle while cutting weight, consider it a bonus.

If you selected the second muscle development goal, you will be focused on increasing your muscle mass while trying to minimize increasing your body fat. This means that you will be dieting to achieve a calorie surplus. Doing this requires consistently eating slightly more calories than you need. Note that eating a nutritious protein rich-diet is just as important when you're trying to gain weight as when you're trying to lose it. Even if your diet is perfect, you will almost certainly gain *some* amount of additional body fat during the muscle-building process. For this reason, closely monitoring body fat is important to ensure that your fat levels don't become unhealthy. Once you're happy with your muscle development, you should consider a brief calorie deficit to remove residual fat that accumulated during the muscle-building process.

If you're aiming to build muscle mass, clearly understanding how much muscle average people are capable of building is important. First, let's talk about what's technically possible, then we'll cover what's realistic for most people. An adult man just beginning with consistent strength training is generally capable of gaining about one to two pounds of muscle mass per month. Adult women can generally gain muscle at about half the rate of a comparable male, so half a pound to one pound per month.[6] Based on these estimated rates, a man could put on a maximum of about twenty-four pounds of muscle in his first year of training. Likewise, a woman could put on a maximum of about twelve pounds of muscle during her first year. Note that people capable of achieving the *maximum* rate of muscle gain must have many factors working in their favor. Having superior genetics, maintaining perfect nutrition, being young, and spending extra time training all can help a person achieve the maximum muscle gains. The average person probably won't gain muscle at the maximum rates because all these stars won't be aligned for them.

How much muscle gain, then, is achievable for the average person who is willing to engage in short twenty-minute daily workouts? In many cases, men with no consistent training history can expect to gain ten pounds or more during their first year. Likewise, many women can set a baseline expectation of developing around five pounds of muscle in their first year. With these estimates given, recognize that they are just broad estimates. You may be someone who's initially capable of building muscle at two pounds per month, or you may be able to develop at a rate of only half a pound per month. Some people are genetically predisposed to developing muscle quickly while others are not. Regardless of your genetics, you *are* capable of building strength and muscle mass with proper diet and training.[7]

At this point you might be wondering, What happens after the first year of consistent training? Can I continue gaining muscle mass at the same rate year after year for a lifetime? The answer is no. Each of us has a certain genetic potential for building muscle, and as you approach it, your capacity to build additional muscle will slow down.[8] Keep this in mind if you're aiming to build a significant amount of muscle mass. Even though your muscle gains will slow and eventually plateau—probably after your first few years—strength training will continue to be vital to your fitness program because *maintaining* muscle mass and strength become more crucial to your quality of life as you age. Also remember that gaining muscle mass requires eating a consistent calorie surplus, so the gaining potentials just described apply only to people who consistently eat enough to build muscle. If you plan to maintain a calorie deficit or energy balance, you won't see significant increases in muscle mass—though you will likely experience some strength gains.

Popular Myths and Misconceptions

Now that you know how to set realistic expectations, let's dispel some popular myths and misconceptions about strength training and body composition. Doing so is important because many of these ideas are widely circulated and believed. To keep them from influencing your training and development expectations, you need to be aware of them and know why they're flawed.

The Neverland Fallacy

Unfortunately, many adults (especially ex-athletes) believe themselves capable of building strength and muscle quickly because they did so as teenagers. They mistakenly credit their past muscle development to exercise programs they followed at the time, which were usually related to sports participation. These people often don't realize that the development they once experienced was aided strongly by the hormonal changes happening in their teenage bodies. When you're a teenager in puberty, your body produces human growth hormone at about double the rate of an adult. This results in muscles being more responsive to training and requiring less time for recovery. For this reason, teens can develop at a faster rate during these years. Even if you did no strength training during puberty, you probably gained about 25 percent of your adult size—including muscle mass—during this short period.[9] Virtually no adult has the potential to gain mass at the same rate as a teenager—not without the aid of pharmaceuticals (steroids). The training that young exercisers and athletes do lends to their muscle growth, but the development they experience is significantly amplified by their elevated hormone levels.

Due to the misconception just described, many people think that as adults, they should exercise in the same way they did in adolescence. A major problem with following your old high school workout routine is that it was probably a sport-specific type of program. This means it was designed for certain athletic results. Adults should generally be exercising to optimize overall health and fitness, not to achieve specialized athletic performance. Another issue with these sport-specific programs is that most are designed for two to four days of training per week. This is a great rhythm for athletes who're balancing practice and competition, but two-to-four-day-per-week programs are not ideal for the average adult trying to make exercise a long-term habit. As you now know, the best prescription for getting stronger, leaner, and more fit is through twenty-minute daily training sessions. Even with consistent training, adults still won't build strength or muscle as quickly as when they were teens because their body chemistry has changed.

To gain muscle, many people also believe that they should eat the same type of diet they followed when they had success in adolescence. Doing so is also a mistake in most cases. As with exercise, teenagers' bodies respond very differently to diet than adults'. The main problem with adults eating like they did as a teenager is that teenagers tend to eat more. This is especially the case with ex–high school athletes, many of whom were consuming three, four, or even five thousand calories a day. While such a high calorie intake makes sense for some athletes, doing so for most adults is a recipe for increased body fat.

The Fat-Conversion Myth

Hearing people talk about the notion of "converting fat into muscle" is quite common. You often hear this said about someone who was overweight and became leaner and more visibly muscular quickly. When people see these transformations happen, many conclude that being overweight is somehow helpful for becoming muscular. They think, If fat can be converted into muscle and I have plenty of fat, then I have more "material" for building strong muscles compared to a thinner person. The error here is that fat and muscle are two completely different types of tissue. The body cannot "transform" fat tissue into muscle.

The idea that fat can be turned into muscle is akin to the popular medieval idea of alchemy—that lead can be converted into gold. Just as modern science debunked the claims of alchemy, it has also debunked the fat-conversion myth. Fat is a passive tissue that basically just stores excess calories for later use. Muscle is an active tissue that expands and contracts, burns calories, and allows our bodies to move.[10] The only way to reduce fat is by burning excess calories. The only way to build muscle is through appropriate exercise and nutrition. As you've already learned, building muscle while also losing weight is difficult because the two processes generally conflict with one another. What's happening when an overweight person achieves significant weight loss and seems to become muscular is that they were *already* muscular. In these cases, their muscle was just hidden beneath a layer of body fat.

The Bulking-Up Myth

Hearing of people (often women) who refrain from strength training because of a fear of getting huge bulky muscles is common. These individuals are averse to the idea of building muscle and are therefore generally averse to the idea of strength training. The problem is that they're conflating the purpose of strength training with the rapid gain of muscle mass. They're also not considering what's required to achieve substantial muscle growth. Significant muscle growth has three main requirements: strength training, a nutritious diet, and a maintained calorie surplus. If someone strength trains and eats healthy but doesn't eat to maintain a surplus, then significant muscle growth isn't going to happen. People who aren't interested in gaining mass should be sticking to a calorie deficit or energy balance diet. If they do so, then they have nothing to worry about, regardless of how much strength training they do. This is the simple rule of thumb for men and women: you won't build bigger muscles unless you're eating to build bigger muscles.

What's ironic about the belief that strength training will cause unwanted mass gain is that the opposite usually happens. Most people who don't exercise are almost certainly going to *lose* weight if they start doing any type of consistent workout—including strength training. This happens because even exercises such as weightlifting cause you to begin steadily burning more calories, even if you make no changes to your diet. This fact should make anyone who believes that strength training causes the gain of tons of bulky muscle to reconsider. Instead of concerning yourself about gaining unwanted muscle, you should be concerned with the very real threat of losing muscle as you age. Strength training is the only known way to prevent natural muscle degeneration, so it should be universally embraced, not avoided.

The Strength-Training-Is-Not-for-Women Myth

Gender plays an interesting role in how people determine their health goals. Likewise, it seems to have a particularly strong influence on how regularly a person engages in strength training. Generally, *all* adults should exercise their major muscle groups two to three times per week, but active men are much more likely to do so than women. According to the US Bureau of Labor Statistics, only 29.7 percent of active women report lifting weights compared to 70.3 percent of men.[11] A likely explanation for this is that women tend to view the value of strength training differently than men, which can be problematic.

The following probably isn't a surprise to you: for most Americans the "ideal" male body is a muscular upper body with a thin waistline; the "ideal" female body type is very slim and lean. This was confirmed in a 2012 British study, which also showed that men and women barely differ in their opinions of these ideal body types. A similar study found that contemporary North American "body ideals" promote strength for men and thinness for women.[12] These gender-specific body ideals seem to play a significant role in determining our health goals and the exercises we select to help achieve them. While the source of these ideal body types is debatable, people should consider how these ideas might be affecting their choices. Specifically, women should consider the health benefits that they might be missing out on while avoiding strength training.

Another potentially negative effect of traditional body ideals relates to people's interest in what others think about them and their desire not to be ostracized. This phenomenon is called *evaluation concern*. A 2010 study hypothesized that evaluation concern is more likely for women in cases where they violate social expectations in their choice of exercise. The study found that weightlifting activities are viewed as much more characteristic of men while engaging in cardio exercise is thought to be more characteristic of women. The hypothesis was confirmed when a significant number of the female participants reported that imagining themselves performing strength training *and* actually performing strength training—especially in public—evoked significant evaluation concerns. The women in this study also seemed to be much more comfortable engaging in exercises commonly associated with the body ideal of their gender (i.e., cardio exercise). Other studies have also shown that women are usually underrepresented among users of free weights and other strength-training equipment.[13]

The seemingly common tendency of women to put less focus on or completely avoid strength training as a means of exercise is concerning for multiple reasons. In addition to the general benefits of strength training, these exercises provide women with many gender-specific health benefits that shouldn't be ignored. Weight-bearing exercise is especially important for postmenopausal women because they are much more susceptible to bone loss. Resistance training helps prevent bone loss and can even build new bone, preventing or lessening the impact of osteoporosis. Some research has also suggested that weight-lifting can have significant psychological benefits. It can provide some-what of a barrier against common psychological conditions in women, such as eating disorders and body dissatisfaction.[14]

The long-standing ideal female form—thin and lean—has been exclusively associated with cardio exercise for far too long. Though there's been an increased popularity of some strength-training pro-grams across genders (such as with CrossFit), this isn't enough. Too many people still believe that doing cardio exclusively is the only way for a woman to get the body she wants. The cultural pressure women feel to steer clear of strength training is a consequence of so many people still clinging to this outdated belief. Resolving this problem requires you to lessen the associations you hold between cardio exer-cise and the ideal female body. Strength training plays a huge role in the development of a physically fit human body, regardless of gender.

Women—or men—who focus only on burning fat via cardio exer-cise will experience muscle loss. If not corrected, losing muscle mass will eventually lead to a loss of strength and mobility and put women at risk for other health issues as they age. Is the cardio-only approach a shortcut to losing weight and staying lean? Yes. Is the long-term effect on a woman's body worth the cost of taking this approach? Absolutely not. In fact, it greatly increases the probability that she'll fail to form a healthy exercise habit, which will almost certainly reduce the quality and length of her life. With the right information, effective tactics, and the desire to get fit, all women healthy enough to exercise should feel confident in adding strength training to their exercise regimen.

The Strength-Training-Is-for-the-Young Myth

The final myth that we'll address is about how a person's age impacts a person's overall fitness for strength training. Hearing people over fifty claim that strength training is not appropriate for them due to their age is common. Culturally, this claim is usually an acceptable excuse, but physiologically, it's simply not true. Most older individuals who hold this idea haven't consulted with a physician to assess their fitness for strength exercises, so they have no idea what physical limitations (if any) they may have. Even in cases of a chronic condition or injury, most doctors won't advise against strength training outright.

While you should consult with a physician if you're in questionable health, there's no general reason that people of any age shouldn't do strength training. In fact, the US Department of Health and Human Services recommends that older adults regularly engage in muscle-strengthening exercises. This broad recommendation stems from a growing body of research that supports activities such as weightlifting for people of all ages. Many clinical trials have shown that even adults in their eighties benefit from strength training, *even* when they have preexisting health conditions.[15] Despite the popular myth about being "too old," the evidence suggests that all people who want a higher quality of life should embrace strength training.

Conclusion

In this chapter, you've learned the basics about how muscle and fat mass are developed and controlled. You've also learned how to set *realistic expectations* about your goal profile.

Your new knowledge and expectations will prepare you to take control of your physique and steer your physical development in the desired direction. The details of how to do this are covered in parts 3 and 4.

CHAPTER 7

Body-Composition Management

WHETHER YOU'VE ACHIEVED YOUR IDEAL body composition or you have a long way to go, you should have a consistent process for monitoring your development, a feedback mechanism that indicates whether your diet and exercise efforts are working. In other words, it should tell you if you're reducing fat, gaining fat, maintaining muscle, gaining muscle, or whatever your goals are. Having a clear line of sight to how your body composition is changing allows you to optimize your training and nutrition plans rapidly and dynamically. This is important because no one's body composition remains totally static; body composition constantly changes due to factors both in and out of our control. The best way to direct these changes in the desired direction is by frequently checking and responding to the small fluctuations in your physical metrics.

Checking Daily Metrics

The three essential metrics that must be regularly checked to effectively manage body composition were introduced in chapter 5: body weight, body-fat percentage, and muscle mass. Those who are serious about being in command of their physique should be checking all three of these indicators daily. Is it possible to get by with checking less frequently? Yes, but the more frequently you check metrics, the more rapidly you can respond to changes. The other benefit of checking daily is that you will psychologically reinforce the relationship between diet, exercise, and your body composition. Observing how your composition changes from day to day is also a great way to learn how your body responds to exercise and nutrition. After just a few months of daily checking, you'll get surprisingly good at understanding how your daily metrics relate to your diet and exercise patterns.

The good news is that creating the daily habit of checking body metrics is easy if you anchor the procedure to your existing morning routine. Most people go to the bathroom right after waking up, so keep your scale and body fat calipers stored in the bathroom. After using the restroom, strip down and hop on the scale to check your weight. After that, grab your calipers and quickly take your body fat measurements. From here, navigate to an FFMI calculator on your smart phone to quickly calculate your FFMI. This whole procedure should just take a few minutes. From here, you can put on your workout gear and head to your home-gym area to knock out your twenty-minute daily workout.

Interpreting Metrics

Now that you know how to make metrics checks a daily habit, next you'll need to learn what these measurements can tell you about your body composition. A changing FFMI indicates that you're gaining or losing muscle, which will cause a change in body weight but not necessarily a change in body fat. Likewise, changes in body-fat percentage mean a change in fat mass and body weight but not necessarily a change in muscularity. Note that your FFMI and body-fat percentage can change without affecting one another, but a change in either causes a change in total body weight. This is because FFMI and body-fat percentage both measure smaller components of your total mass, but body weight measures your total mass.

Knowing how to interpret your body metrics allows you to assess how your fitness program is changing your physique. For instance, the first question to ask yourself upon seeing an increase in body weight is, What is the source of the weight gain—a gain in muscle or fat? To answer this question, you should look at how your FFMI and body-fat percentage have been trending to determine the main source of the weight gain. Let's assume that your goal is to increase muscle mass and maintain body fat. If you found that the weight gain came from an increased FFMI, then you would have made progress toward your goal. If you found that the weight gain came mainly from an increase in body fat, then you wouldn't have made progress toward your goal.

Below are more examples of the types of conclusions that could be drawn by tracking and analyzing your key metrics over time. For each example, assume that the individual's body weight, body-fat percentage, and FFMI are being checked daily.

- Anthony's total weight increased by five pounds. His FFMI has increased, but his body-fat percentage has remained the same. Conclusion: Anthony has gained five pounds of muscle.
- Lauren's total weight has increased by ten pounds. Her FFMI has not changed but her fat percentage has increased. Conclusion: Lauren has gained ten pounds of fat.
- Charles lost ten pounds of body weight, but his FFMI stayed the same. Conclusion: Charles has lost ten pounds of fat.
- Angela lost ten pounds of body weight. Her FFMI and body-fat percentage have both dropped. Conclusion: Angela has lost a combination of muscle and fat. (To calculate specifically how many pounds of fat is lost versus muscle, subtract previous lean

body mass from current lean body mass, which will indicate the amount of muscle mass lost. Then subtract muscle lost from the total amount of weight lost to calculate fat loss.)

After you've learned to interpret body-composition metrics, you'll be able to determine what adjustments to your fitness program might be needed. For example, Chad occasionally allows himself to eat foods outside of his normal diet, which results in a calorie surplus. The impact of these surpluses is evident during his daily metrics checks in the form of slightly increased weight and body fat. His reaction to these body mass changes are to moderately reduce his normal calorie intake for a few days until his metrics return to the desired levels.

As another example, Alicia is trying to reduce her body fat but notices a significant decrease in her FFMI over several days—indicating a loss of muscle mass. This likely means her calorie deficit is too extreme and needs to be adjusted. It may also mean she's not challenging her muscles with enough resistance during exercise (more on this in chapters 8 and 9). Notice that in both examples, changes in key metrics are the primary indicator that changes need to be made to the person's fitness program.

Maintaining a Metrics Record

A critical part of metrics checks is documenting your daily results. Documenting is important because you won't be capable of remembering your past metrics over the course of multiple days. If you try to rely on memory, you'll end up making decisions about your fitness program based on day-to-day fluctuations in your metrics. This can be a problem because in many cases, you need to see the long-term trends in your development to make good fitness decisions. Making the wrong decisions about diet and exercise makes achieving your goals difficult and may cause you to lose motivation. To identify the long-term trends, you'll need to see the documented history of your body-composition metrics. These trends will give a clearer picture of your overall trajectory and will often influence your goals for the better.

Let's look at an example of how drawing conclusions and making fitness decisions based solely on day-to-day metrics changes can be a problem. Jordan is trying to lose some body fat. He works an irregular nightshift schedule, so the times of day that he sleeps, exercises, and eats meals can vary widely. When you eat, how much you've slept, and when you work out can all influence metrics readings, especially body weight. These factors can make it difficult to interpret the meaning of changes in your metrics from one day to the next. Due to this, Jordan often sees his daily weight fluctuate erratically—even though he's sticking to his fitness plan. By just assessing the day-to-day changes in his metrics, he can easily conclude that his pursuit of better fitness is failing. The problem is that often irregular sleep, eating, and workout schedules are the main cause of fluctuations in body metrics. In other words, Jordan could be improving his body composition without it being evident in his day-to-day metrics checks.

How can you tell if you're making progress when day-to-day metrics changes don't indicate success? How do you identify the longer-term trends? The best solution is to calculate and compare weekly, every two weeks, or even monthly averages. In many cases, looking for trends across larger timescales can tell a different story about your progress. Table 6.1 shows how a weight loss trend, for instance, can be seen by comparing week-to-week averages. Note that taking averages is a good strategy for any body metric—body weight, body fat percent, and FFMI.

Table 6.1

An Example of Weight Loss Trends with Weekly Averages

Week 1	Weight	Week 2	Weight	Week 3	Weight	Week 4	Weight
1/1	164.7	1/8	164.2	1/15	164.1	1/22	163.2
1/2	165.2	1/9	163.6	1/16	163.3	1/23	163.1
1/3	164.4	1/10	164.4	1/17	163.2	1/24	163.5
1/4	165	1/11	164.1	1/18	163.4	1/25	163
1/5	164.1	1/12	164.2	1/19	164.1	1/26	163.4
1/6	165.1	1/13	163.8	1/20	163.4	1/27	163.1
1/7	164.6	1/14	164.2	1/21	163.7	1/28	163.3
Weekly averages	164.7		164.1		163.6		163.2
Average weight loss from previous week	0		0.6 lb		0.5 lb		0.4 lb

Using averages to see longer-term trends isn't just a solution for those with an irregular schedule, this solution is helpful in many scenarios. For example, when you're close to achieving a goal and just need to lose that last pound of fat. Anytime you think you're not making progress, validate that conclusion by looking at the averages over longer periods of time.

Now you're probably wondering, What's the best way to log my daily numbers? You can create a metrics log in many ways. The most important step is to capture the three key measurements for each day *and* the date of those measurements. Below are a few good ideas for creating your own body composition log:

- Create a spreadsheet with a separate column for weight, body-fat percentage, FFMI, and date. The benefit of spreadsheets is that they can easily calculate averages and help identify trends.
- Use a paper notebook or journal to capture each daily measurement.
- Use the notes application on your smart phone.

Pick the option that works best for you, and create your log!

Long–Term Body–Composition Management

A common question at this point is, How long do I need to maintain my body composition log? Simple answer: it should be a lifelong fitness habit. Most people only keep track of metrics such as body weight when they're trying to achieve a short-term goal, for example losing five or ten pounds. Once they've lost the weight, they tend to stop tracking their metrics because they believe that the work is done once they become "fit." This is a massive mistake that will probably lead to a body you're unhappy with.

The secret that perpetually fit people understand is that fitness is not something that you arrive at. Fitness is an ongoing process, which is most easily maintained by building efficient and effective habits. Even the most fit people must make little tweaks and adjustments to their process to keep them where they want to be. Just like you, their body compositions fluctuate. They're just able to react to and correct the small fluctuations quickly and easily—so their composition changes are less noticeable. They know how to react to unwanted changes by first knowing their key body measurements. Your body composition will always require attention and management, and doing this becomes easy when checking and logging your key metrics is a daily habit.

Many fitness programs and gurus advocate *not* measuring and tracking body composition regularly because it can cause stress or anxiety. This is not the best approach for most people. If you have a long way to go on your fitness journey, you won't make progress by *not* observing the physical facts. If taking body measurements causes you stress or anxiety, the proper way to alleviate those issues is by confronting the facts and developing a plan of action. You won't achieve your long-term goals overnight, but you will build confidence in yourself by making *any degree* of progress. When you see yourself systematically making progress, you don't have to feel anxious or stressed—you can feel proud.

This simple analogy sums up why measuring and tracking body composition is a requirement: winning the game is harder when you don't know the score. Think of your body-composition log as a scoreboard. It tells you when you're winning and warns you when you're falling behind. When you check the scoreboard often, you'll know when to change your plays. This allows you to deal with problems when they're small rather than letting them compound into larger issues.

Conclusion

In this chapter, you learned why checking body weight, body-fat percentage, and muscle mass regularly is important and why checking these metrics daily is best. You now know the most efficient ways to measure these metrics and how to integrate those practices into your daily routine. You've also learned how to interpret your body-composition metrics to determine the effectiveness of your fitness program. By tracking daily metrics in a log, you'll be able to monitor your body composition over time and identify trends that will help you draw more accurate conclusions about your progress—which is critical to determining when program adjustments might be needed. If you can make the simple procedures described in this chapter into a habit, you'll be instituting a powerful feedback mechanism that will serve as the primary compass on your lifelong fitness journey.

PART 3

~~~~~

The Nuts and Bolts of Exercise

Part 3 is all about the types of exercise you should do and how to arrange your exercises into an effective workout program. It covers the following topics:

- Six essential types of strength-training exercises and how to do them at home
- Selecting appropriate ab and cardio exercises
- How to group your various exercises into short twenty-minute workouts
- Tips and tricks for recovery, selecting appropriate rep and set volumes, adjusting weight and resistance levels, gauging your heart rate, and tracking progress

By the end of this section, you'll have the knowledge required to select your preferred exercises, assess your equipment needs, design your routine, and most importantly, begin the process of building your lifelong exercise habit.

Note that the scope and purpose of this section is to educate people about some of the most common and widely used exercise options that can be efficiently incorporated into a low-friction routine. Though it does provide general recommendations about certain exercises that can be highly effective, it does so only for educational purposes. These exercises may not be appropriate for everyone. If you don't have adequate prior experience with exercise or aren't certain of your ability to perform the exercises described safely and correctly, then consulting with an exercise professional prior to starting a new exercise routine is advisable. If you have reason to believe that you're not healthy enough for the types of exercises described, you should consult with your physician or other qualified healthcare professional prior to starting a new routine.

CHAPTER 8

~~~〜〜

Strength‑Training
Fundamentals

ANYONE WHO'S EVER ATTEMPTED TO develop a workout plan on his or her own knows how challenging it can be. One of the most difficult parts is determining the right types of individual exercises to do—which is especially true when it comes to strength training. Most people generally don't have the knowledge or time to figure this out, which is why they opt for readymade exercise programs. The problem with most readymade strength programs is that they're not specifically designed to minimize friction and optimize the use of your time and energy. This chapter lays the groundwork for building a custom work‑out plan by highlighting the most important details needed to choose the best strength-training exercises.

To pick the right exercises, you should consider only those that provide the maximum amount of benefit in the least amount of time. In other words, you need to choose the most efficient exercises. Taking this approach results in short and effective workouts that will mini‑mize friction in your life. Before we jump in, note that what consti‑tutes an efficient strength exercise is different from what constitutes efficient cardio. This chapter focuses exclusively on helping you select the most appropriate strength-training exercises for your daily workouts. Chapter 9 will cover the selection of efficient cardio exercises.

Defining Efficient Strength-Training Exercises

To select the most efficient strength exercises, identify the ones that engage the highest number of important muscles all in one movement. When you pick exercises that do this, you'll work more muscles with fewer exercises and in less time. Doing so results in a less complicated exercise program with shorter workouts. Taking this approach is an important shortcut because strength training is inherently more complicated than cardio.

Cardio is less complicated because its primary goal is to work only one muscle, the heart, which only requires one type of exercise. Full-body strength training requires regularly working all your major muscle groups—your legs, chest, back, shoulders, arms, and midsection. Working these various muscles requires doing several types of exercises. The following few sections will help you cut through the complexity of strength training by teaching you to select the most effective strength exercises.

What Are Compound Exercises?

The strength exercises that work the greatest number of important muscles in one movement are called *compound exercises*. Some common examples are the squat, dead lift, and bench press. Compound exercises require you to use multiple joints to exert force against resistance. Using multiple joints allows you to exert more force than during isolation—single-joint—exercises such as biceps curls, triceps extensions, and leg curls. Exerting more force is critical because it allows you to push or pull against more resistance, which is ideal for developing and maintaining muscle mass.[1]

Despite the multitude of fad workout programs that come and go, virtually all of them rely on compound exercises. This is the case because compound exercises are effective, which is why they've been central to competitive strength training since its beginnings. Lifts such as snatches and presses were some of the first events in the nineteenth-century Olympics, and their roots go all the way back to ancient Greece and Egypt.[2] Keep this in mind the next time you're tempted by a new exercise craze. No matter what workout fad comes next, one truth won't change: getting stronger and developing muscle requires lifting heavy stuff, which can only be done effectively and safely in a few ways.

The Essential Compound Exercises

Here are the six most essential compound movements that must be part of your exercise program:

- Horizontal push (or press)
- Horizontal pull
- Vertical push
- Vertical pull
- Hip-dominant pull
- Quad-dominant push[3]

While other compound lifts exist that use even more muscles at once (e.g., snatches, cleans, jerks), they tend to be more complicated movements. These lifts tend to require advanced technique and have a greater risk of injury. The exercise types listed above are relatively simple to learn and execute. You will be able to perform them after some basic instruction, even if you've never done them before. Overall, these six types of motion will give the best balance of effectiveness, simplicity, and safety for your workouts.

The following sections describe the essential compound movements and advise how to select the right exercises to include in your workout program. Please note that this book is not intended to be an exhaustive guide on exercise technique. If you need more specific instructions on technique, try one of the following options:

- Search for professional demonstrations on the internet.
- Buy a book on exercise technique.
- Temporarily hire a licensed coach or trainer.

The Horizontal Push

The horizontal push is a compound-exercise type that focuses on large muscle groups in the chest, shoulders, and upper back—such as the pectorals, triceps, deltoids, and trapezius (trap) muscles. All horizontal pushes primarily use the arms, shoulders, and chest muscles to exert force forward, away from the torso. The most common type of horizontal push is the bench press and its many variations, but other exercises fall into this category, such as dumbbell presses, machine presses, and push-ups.[4] Most types of horizontal push do require some equipment:

- A bench press and set of dumbbells
- A bench press and barbell set
- A machine press of some kind

For the average person working out in a home gym, sticking with a traditional bench press or dumbbell press is best, as shown in figures 8.1 and 8.2.

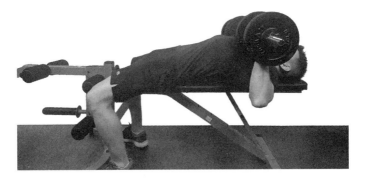

Figure 8.1: Dumbbell bench press down

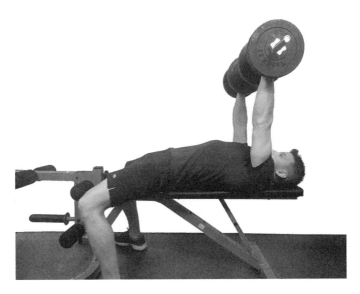

Figure 8.2: Dumbbell bench press up

The only exception would be for those with an injury or other physical limitation that makes these impossible. In these cases, you can consider an alternative. Note the traditional bench press does require a spotter to be performed safely, but you can easily solve this problem. The best option is purchasing a weight bench and separate weightlifting rack of some kind—weight racks have safety mechanisms that serve as a spotter so you can lift safely without a partner. Never perform the traditional bench press alone if you don't have some type of safety spotter.

Many types of weightlifting racks are available, such as squat racks, squat stands, and power racks. Here are the most important factors to consider when selecting a weightlifting rack:

- Does it have some type of safety spotter mechanism? It should.
- Can you easily move a weight bench in and out of the rack? This is important because for some other exercises, you'll want to move your bench away from the rack. (Purchasing racks that have benches permanently attached to them is usually not ideal. Doing so will ultimately require you to buy a separate bench for other exercises.)
- Will the rack fit in your home-gym space? Some racks take up minimal space while others are quite large. Select one with a footprint that works for your situation.
- Does the rack have a pull-up bar? Many do, and this is a nice addition because it eliminates the need to buy separate equipment for vertical pull exercises.

Figures 8.3 and 8.4 show examples of a good bench press setup.

Chest press machines of all kinds are also safe options if you have the money and space for them. If you're wary of purchasing a bench press or machine, you can temporarily stick to push-ups or purchase an adjustable set of resistance bands. Resistance bands can provide all the resistance necessary for an effective chest press, as shown in figures 8.5 and 8.6. They are relatively inexpensive, and they take up no space.

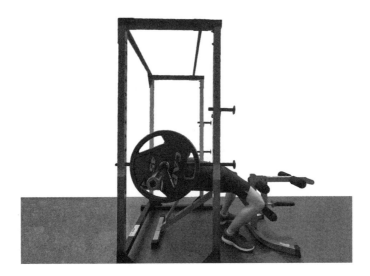

Figure 8.3: Bench press down

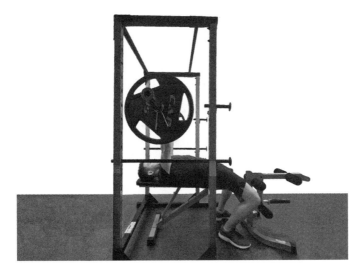

Figure 8.4: Bench press up

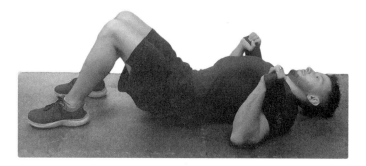

Figure 8.5: Resistance band press down

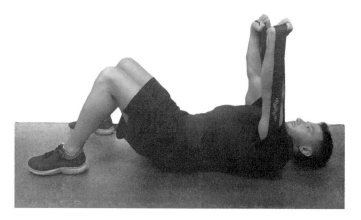

Figure 8.6: Resistance band press up

The Horizontal Pull

The horizontal pull is a type of compound exercise that primarily focuses on the large muscles of the back, such as the latissimus dorsi (lats), rhomboids, and traps; they also work the biceps. These motions primarily use the upper back and arms to pull against resistance directly toward the torso. The most common type of horizontal pull is the row, which has many different variations, such as T-bar rows, bent-over rows, seated cable rows, and machine rows.[5] Most of these exercises require some equipment, but having just a flat bench and a barbell or dumbbell set will give you multiple options.

One-arm dumbbell rows are the best option for most people, as shown in figures 8.7 and 8.8. They are done by bending over a flat bench and supporting yourself with one hand and knee on the bench. The opposite leg is planted on the floor, and the free hand holds the weighted dumbbell and executes the pulling motion toward the torso. This version of the row keeps your body extremely stable and has a low risk of injury. If the weight is too heavy, you can simply set it on the floor or let it drop.

If you need an alternative that requires less equipment, adjustable resistance bands are an easy solution, as shown in figures 8.9 and 8.10. A horizontal rowing motion can be done many ways using bands.

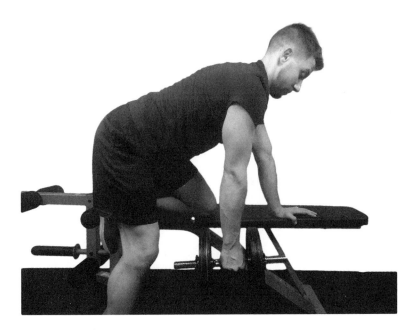

Figure 8.7: Dumbbell row down

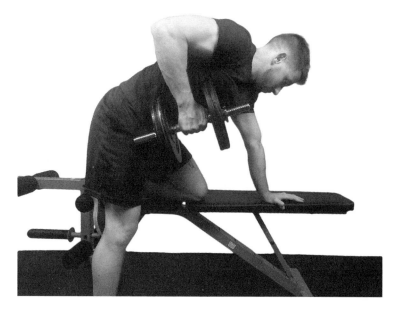

Figure 8.8: Dumbbell row up

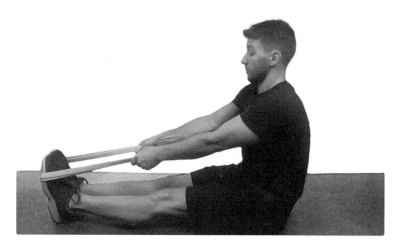

Figure 8.9: Resistance band row down

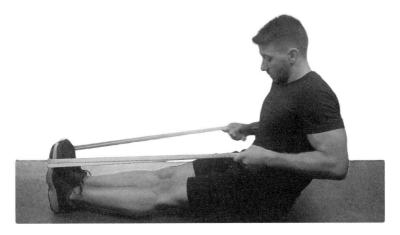

Figure 8.10: Resistance band row up

The Vertical Push

The vertical push is a compound-exercise type that focuses on the shoulder muscles but also works some chest and arm muscles. Specifically, this exercise works the deltoids (delts), upper chest, and triceps. All these exercises use the arms and shoulders to exert force in an upward, overhead motion against resistance. Some common exercises in this category are standing military presses, dumbbell presses, single-arm presses, seated shoulder presses, and high-incline bench presses.[6] Most of these exercises can be done with either a barbell set or dumbbells. The seated types can be done on an adjustable bench placed in the upright position; some can even be done in a regular chair. Many types of shoulder-press machines are also available for those with the space and budget. The benefit of a machine is a reduced risk of injury due to increased stability.

The seated shoulder press using dumbbells is the best option for most people, as shown in figures 8.11 and 8.12. Here again, the beauty of dumbbells is that they can be set down or safely dropped if they're too heavy. A shoulder press motion can also be performed using resistance bands, as shown in figures 8.13 and 8.14.

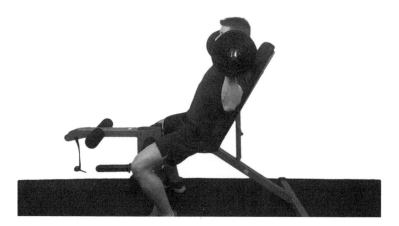

Figure 8.11: Dumbbell shoulder press down

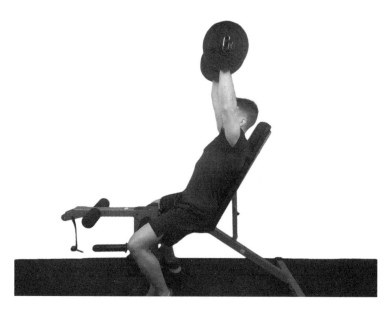

Figure 8.12: Dumbbell shoulder press up

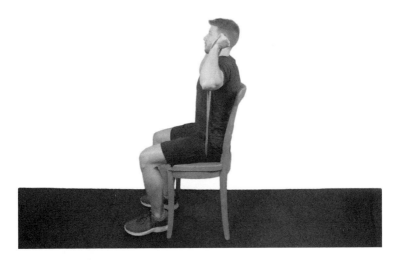

Figure 8.13: Resistance band shoulder press down

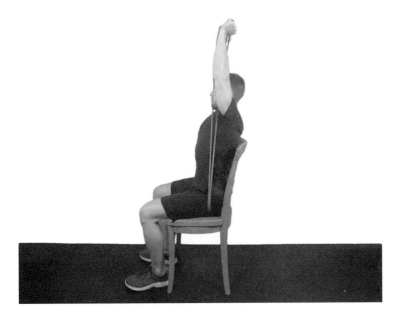

Figure 8.14: Resistance band shoulder press up

If traditional weights are not an option for you, a body weight–only shoulder press known as a pike shoulder press, as shown in figures 8.15 and 8.16, is a good solution. The pike press is performed much like a push-up but with the body bent at a ninety-degree angle with the buttocks elevated high above the head.

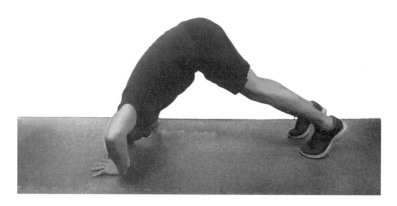

Figure 8.15: Pike press down

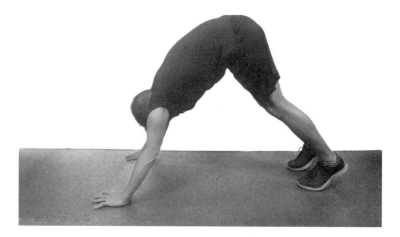

Figure 8.16: Pike press up

The Vertical Pull

The vertical pull is a compound-exercise type that focuses on various muscle groups in your back and arms. It generally works the lats, rhomboids, shoulder joints, and either the biceps or triceps depending on the specific exercise. All vertical pulls involve pulling against resistance from overhead and downward vertically in relation to your torso. The most common vertical pull exercises are chin-ups (which are biceps dominant), pull-ups (which are triceps dominant), and lateral pull-downs (which can be biceps or triceps dominant).[7] Pull-ups, chin-ups, and resistance-band pull-downs are usually the easiest vertical pulls to do at home.

Remember that many weightlifting racks already come with integrated pull-up bars (as shown in figures 8.17 and 8.18)—and others have optional pull-up bar attachments instead—making racks a great option in many cases. An extremely inexpensive alternative to weight racks is purchasing a pull-up bar that can be installed in a doorway.

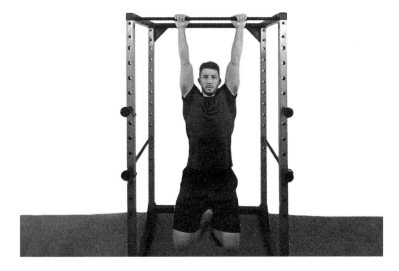

Figure 8.17: Pull-up down

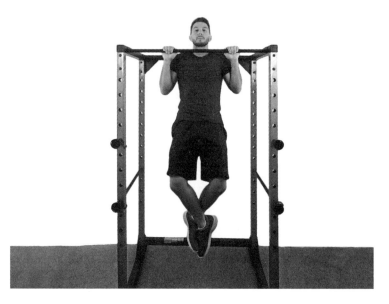

Figure 8.18: Pull-up up

Other types of vertical pulls such as lateral pull-downs can require special machines, which can be expensive and take up significant space.

Choose a biceps-dominant exercise if you prefer doing only one form of vertical pull. However, adding a triceps-dominant vertical pull to your routine can be beneficial.

Chin-ups are depicted in figures 8.19 and 8.20. The steps for executing both pull-ups and chin-ups are as follows:

1. Stand beneath a bar and grab it with your hands—roughly shoulder width apart. Your palms should be facing away from you for pull-ups and toward you for chin-ups.
2. Hang from the bar with arms fully extended and one leg crossed over the other.
3. Pull up against the resistance of your body weight until your chin is level with the bar.[8]

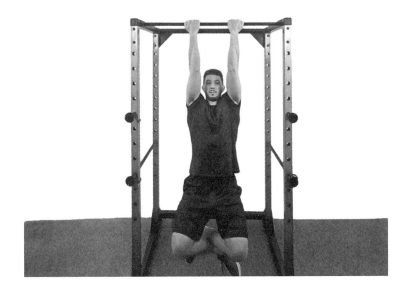

Figure 8.19: Chin-up down

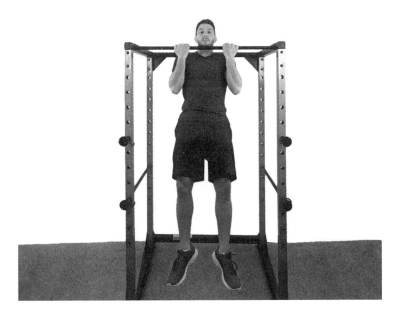

Figure 8.20: Chin-up up

If you don't have the strength for full pull-ups or chin-ups, you can reduce the difficulty by pushing off a chair or other stable surface with one foot. You can also use resistance bands to do assisted vertical pulls. See an example of an assisted vertical pull in figures 8.21 and 8.22.

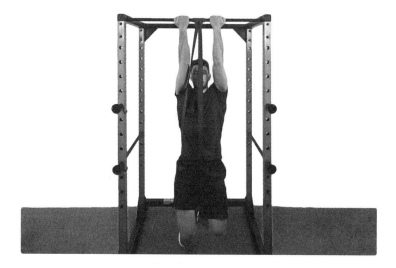

Figure 8.21: Resistance band chin-up down

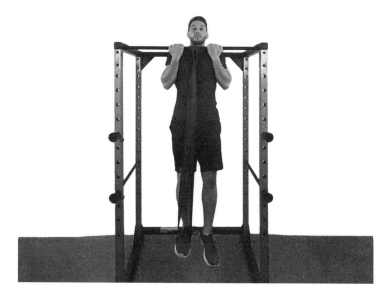

Figure 8.22: Resistance band chin-up up

For those that need an additional challenge beyond their body weight, you can do a weighted version of the pull-up and chin-up. To do this, just put a weighted dumbbell between your feet or thighs to increase the difficulty.

If you need an alternative to pull-ups and chin-ups, you can easily do vertical pull-downs with resistance bands, as shown in figures 8.23, 8.24, 8.25, and 8.26. To do this, mount the bands into a doorway, position yourself beneath it, and perform the pull-down from the floor. Most band sets come with a doorway attachment for this purpose.

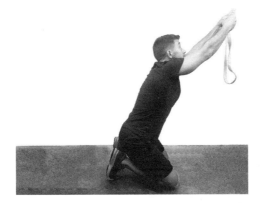

Figure 8.23: Resistance band biceps-dominant pull-down up

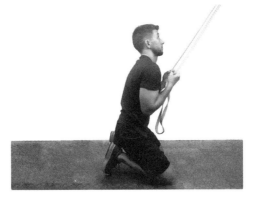

Figure 8.24: Resistance band biceps-dominant pull-down down

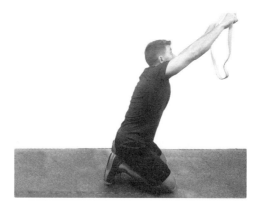

Figure 8.25: Resistance band triceps-dominant pull-down up

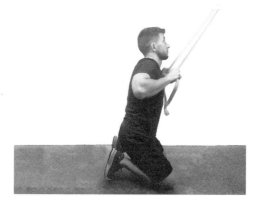

Figure 8.26: Resistance band triceps-dominant pull-down down

The Hip-Dominant Pull

Hip-dominant compound exercises focus on the large muscles in your lower body, primarily the gluteal muscles (glutes) and hamstrings.[9] The most common hip-dominant exercises are dead lifts, but hip extensions are another option. The traditional dead lift and its many variations are popular because of their overall effectiveness. They only require basic free weights to perform, so you don't generally need specialized equipment to do them at home. A dead lift basically requires bending over, grabbing a barbell or dumbbells off the floor, and safely standing up with the weight using the hips and back muscles. Dead lifts can also be done using resistance bands instead of traditional weights—this is an especially great option when you're traveling. The basic steps for the traditional barbell dead lift, shown in figures 8.27, 8.28, and 8.29, are as follows:

1. Stand with your feet slightly wider than shoulder width with your toes under the barbell.
2. Squat down while leaning forward slightly and grab the bar with a shoulder-width grip.
3. Keeping your chest sticking out and head in line with your spine, start the lift by pushing through your heels.
4. Stand up with the weight while keeping the bar close to your body.
5. Finish the lift by squeezing the glutes and pushing your hips slightly forward toward the bar.
6. Slowly lower the weight down to the floor while hinging at the hips.[10]

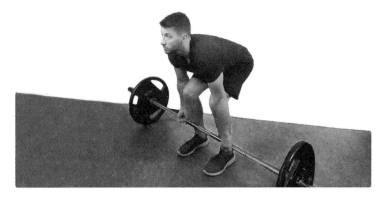

Figure 8.27: Barbell dead lift down

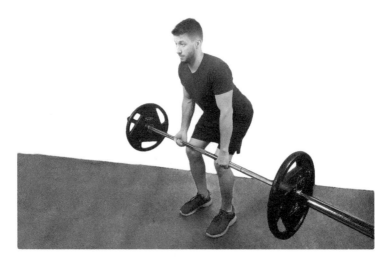

Figure 8.28: Barbell dead lift mid

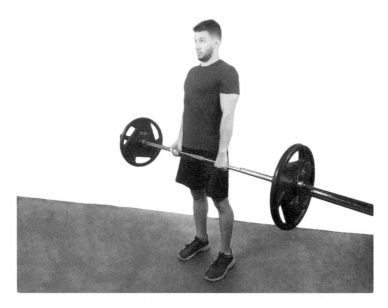

Figure 8.29: Barbell dead lift up

A dumbbell variation, shown in figures 8.30-32, is available as well.

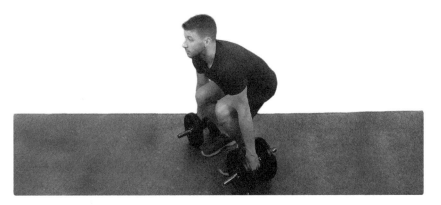

Figure 8.30: Dumbbell dead lift down

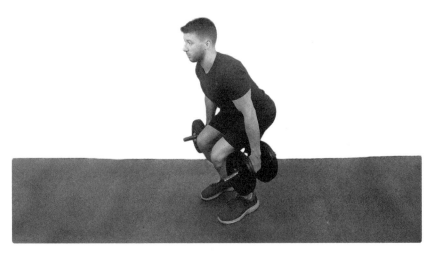

Figure 8.31: Dumbbell dead lift mid

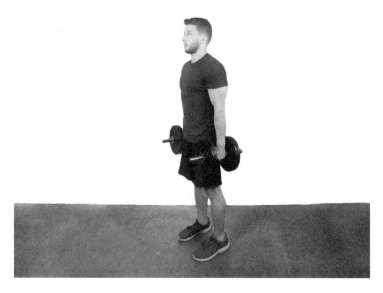

Figure 8.32: Dumbbell dead lift up

You can also use resistance bands, as shown in figures 8.33 and 8.34.

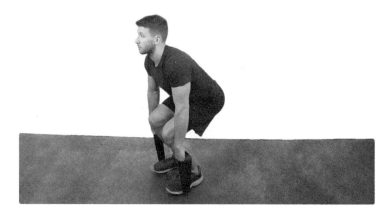

Figure 8.33: Resistance band dead lift down

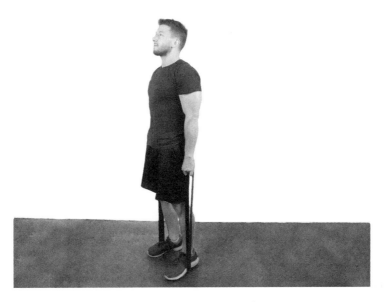

Figure 8.34: Resistance band dead lift up

The best hip-dominant pulling exercise for the average person is the traditional dead lift. If you have knee issues, you can do the Romanian dead lift, which is a straight-legged version of the dead lift that doesn't require bending your knees (shown in figures 8.35 and 8.36).

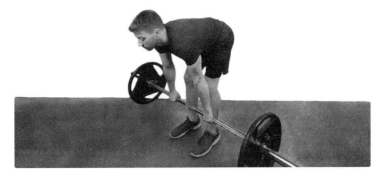

Figure 8.35: Straight-leg dead lift down

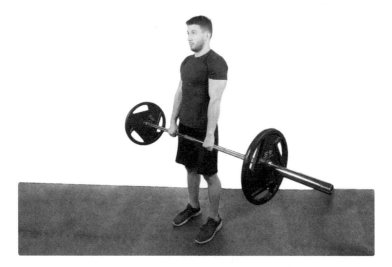

Figure 8.36: Straight-leg dead lift up

With any dead lift, proper technique is critical for preventing injury and ensuring exercise effectiveness. Put special focus on learning to perform this motion properly. Even with proper technique, there's some risk of injury with a dead lift—particularly back injury. If you have back issues or don't want to take the risk, hip extensions (e.g., hyperextensions or back extensions) are a great alternative. They help reduce the risk of injury while still being an effective compound lift.

To do hip extensions at home, you need a hyperextension bench, which is an inclined bench with stabilizers to hold your ankles in place when bent over at the hip so you don't fall heels over head. These benches can often be purchased for less than one hundred dollars, and most are relatively small. People generally think of hip extensions as an exercise done without weights, but they are an effective strength workout when done with them.

Both weighted and nonweighted extensions start with lying face down on the bench with ankles locked in place. You then lean forward—bending at the hip—until the body is at about a ninety-degree angle. From this position you can grab dumbbells (see figures 8.37

and 8.38), a weight plate, or even a barbell (see figures 8.39 and 8.40) that's been positioned on the floor. You then raise the torso back up by thrusting the hip muscles forward and lifting with the lower back, all while keeping your back straight. The motion is complete when the torso has extended fully and is at a straight 180-degree angle with the legs.

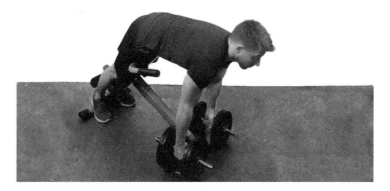

Figure 8.37: Dumbbell back extension down

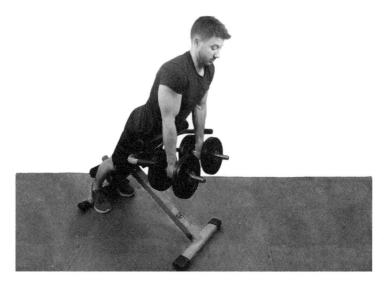

Figure 8.38: Dumbbell back extension up

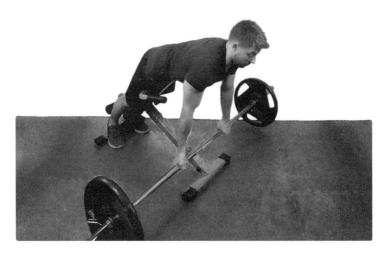

Figure 8.39: Barbell back extension down

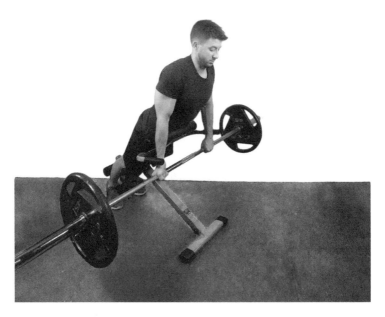

Figure 8.40: Barbell back extension up

The Quad-Dominant Push

Quad-dominant exercises primarily focus on the quadriceps muscles but also work the glutes, hamstrings, and many small stabilizing muscles in the legs.[11] The most popular quad exercise is the squat, but other effective options include lunges, barbell hack squats, leg press (machine), and Smith machine squats. Many quad exercises require special equipment, but you can do effective quad work with just a barbell or set of dumbbells.

The best option for the average person who'll be exercising at home is doing *weighted lunges*. Lunges are an effective compound lift, they're very safe, and they don't require specialized equipment. They are generally done with dumbbells or kettle bells.

The basic steps of a lunge (also shown in figures 8.41 and 8.42) are as follows:

1. Stand upright with your feet together and hold a weight in each hand.
2. Take a big step forward with one leg, leaving the other stationary. In this position, keep the hips and torso upright. This is the starting position.
3. Lower your hips and torso by allowing your forward knee to bend until your thigh is parallel with the floor. As this is happening, your back knee will descend downward until your lower leg becomes roughly parallel to the floor.
4. Complete the lift by pushing with the upper leg muscles of your forward leg to elevate your hips and torso back up to the starting position.
5. Repeat this motion for the desired number of repetitions. Alternate your legs with the lunge to work both legs.[12]

If you need to stop for any reason during a lunge, you can simply drop the weights—which makes this safer than traditional squats.

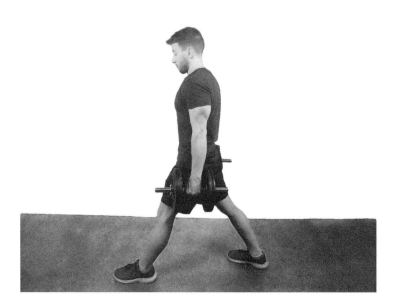

Figure 8.41: Dumbbell lunge up

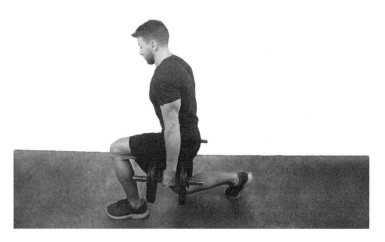

Figure 8.42: Dumbbell lunge down

The leg press machine is another great option for home gyms. It mimics the general squat motion—allowing the lifter to push a significant amount of weight—but in a comparatively safe and controlled manner. The main drawback of this exercise is that the machines are usually expensive and take up quite a bit of space.

The best option when traveling or for those who prefer not to purchase traditional equipment is to perform squats using resistance bands (see figures 8.43 and 8.44). Here's a brief explanation of how to do squats with bands:

1. Start from the standing position with arms raised and supporting the fully extended bands at about shoulder level.
2. While bearing the full resistance of the bands, lower your hips and torso by bending your knees until they reach about a 90-degree angle—be sure to angle your back slightly forward during this motion.
3. Now, push against the resistance with the upper leg muscles to straighten the legs and raise the hips and torso back up to the standing upright position.[13]

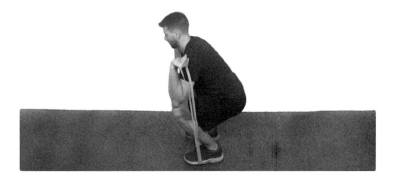

Figure 8.43: Resistance band squat down

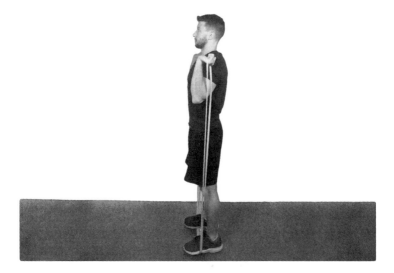

Figure 8.44: Resistance band squat up

Conclusion

In this chapter, you learned which types of strength-training exercises are best for (safely) maximizing your time and energy. You now know that compound exercises are ideal for eliminating friction because they work the greatest number of muscles in one movement. You've also learned about the six essential types of compound movements (horizontal push, horizontal pull, vertical push, vertical pull, hip-dominant pull, and quad-dominant push) and various exercise options for each. By assessing all the options and taking your own preferences, physical abilities and limitations, and home-gym layout into account, you'll be in a good position to select the right strength-training exercises in your workout program. Hold off on making any exercise selections until you've finished reading chapter 9, which explains other important factors that could affect your final choices.

CHAPTER 9

∽꩜

Isolation Exercises, Cardio, and Exercise Selection

NOW THAT YOU KNOW THE importance of the six essential compound strength movements, you need to learn about the other essential types of exercise that should be part of your low-friction program. To help, this chapter explores the following types of exercises:

- Isolation (single joint)
- Abdominal
- Cardiovascular (cardio)

After considering and making recommendations for each, the chapter teaches you how to make smart exercise selections based on your available space, budget, equipment, and personal preferences.

Isolation Exercises

Regularly doing the compound exercise movements described in chapter 8 is essential to efficiently working your major muscle groups. While considering which ones to include in your program, you might wonder if any isolation, or single-joint, exercises should also be included. The answer is that most isolation exercises, such as toe presses or leg curls, aren't necessary for the average person. Body-builders, athletes, and fitness enthusiasts do them because they often have unique goals that require more focused attention on specific muscles. They're willing to spend more time and energy developing these areas because of their specialized performance needs—which aren't a priority for most people.

In general, the essential six types of compound movements will work all the major muscle groups, including those that are commonly thought to require isolation work. For instance, many people believe that they should spend time doing several biceps exercises, such as standing barbell curls and preacher curls, but compound exercises such as rows and chin-ups also work the biceps. Many people also believe that significant time must be spent on triceps exercises such as triceps extensions and pull-downs, but the bench press works the triceps. Overall, the essential compound exercise movements will adequately work your major muscle groups and allow you to build strength and lean muscle mass. If you choose to do any isolation exercises, just know that they will make your workouts longer, which means that exercising will create more friction in your daily routine.

The Case for Ab Exercises

The one type of isolation exercise that you should seriously consider are those that target the abdominal and core muscles. Though many compound exercises, such as the squat and dead lift, engage your core, a strong case can be made for doing some type of isolated core work because these midsection muscles help protect and stabilize your spine. Some people believe that core work isn't necessary, and while certain individuals might be able to get away with no core exercise, doing

ISOLATION EXERCISES, CARDIO, AND EXERCISE SELECTION | 151

something for your abs and core to help prevent injury is advisable.

Selecting the right core exercises can be tricky because no one exercise works all the core muscles. Countless options are available, but some are better than others. What are the best exercises for those who want to use their time and energy efficiently? If you do no other core exercise, the good old-fashioned abdominal crunch is a clear winner. Despite all the available ab machines, novel equipment, and the numerous exotic yoga poses that are now in vogue, a 2014 study done by the American Council on Exercise showed that no exercise elicits more overall abdominal muscle activation than the ab crunch.[1] The big trick with the crunch is that it must be done with the proper technique. The steps for doing a crunch, also shown in figures 9.1 and 9.2, are as follows:

1. Lie on your back with your knees bent and your feet flat on the floor.
2. With your hands behind your head and your chin tucked toward your chest, flex your core muscles while using them to pull your torso toward your thighs—exhale while doing this.
3. As you perform the motion, your upper back should raise slightly off the ground while your lower back remains flat.
4. Briefly hold this position and then uncurl your core muscles while inhaling and returning to the starting position.[2]

Crunches should be performed just like any other strength exercise. When most people think of crunches, they imagine doing twenty-five, fifty, or even one hundred repetitions with just their body weight. Instead, you should do the same number of sets and repetitions for crunches as you do with your compound strength exercises.[3] For instance, if you're doing three sets of ten repetitions for all your compound movements, you should also do three sets of ten crunches.

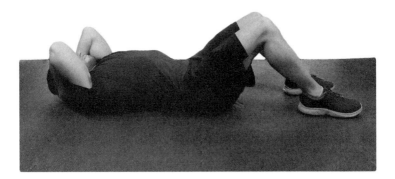

Figure 9.1: Crunch down

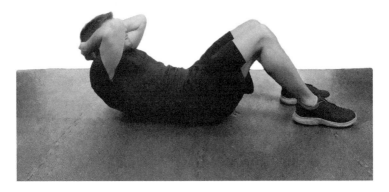

Figure 9.2: Crunch up

When body-weight crunches become too easy, start holding weighted dumbbells over your head while executing crunches to make them more challenging. See an example of the weighted crunch variation in figures 9.3 and 9.4.

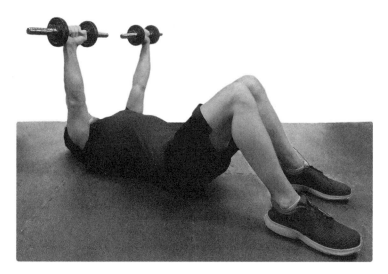

Figure 9.3: Weighted crunch down

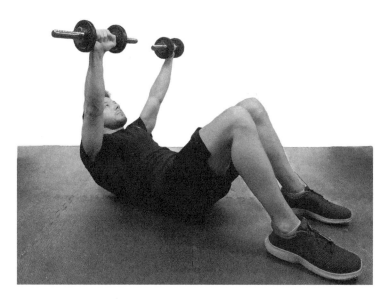

Figure 9.4: Weighted crunch up

Often, people are also curious about the core muscles on their sides called obliques. Folks in yoga and Pilates studios commonly do all sorts of plank exercises to specifically target these muscles. The reality is that traditional crunches engage the external obliques more than front and side planks. Abdominal crunches done properly and with a challenging level of resistance can be all you need to work the critical core muscles. If you want an additional challenge beyond the crunch, a crunch variation called the decline bench curl-up, shown in figures 9.5 and 9.6, is a great option. Essentially, this is just a traditional crunch but performed on a weightlifting bench set in the decline position. This exercise provides all the benefits of the crunch and can be done with or without weights. Plus, it engages the external obliques a bit more.[4]

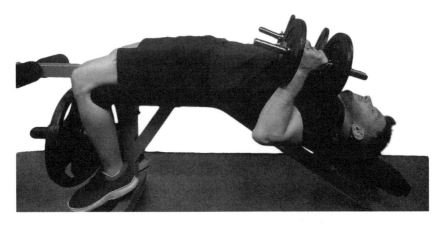

Figure 9.5: Decline curl-up down

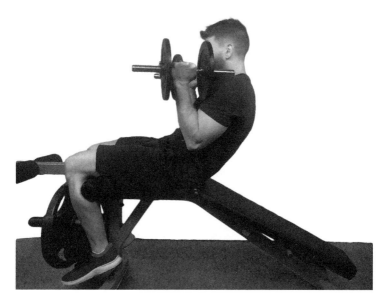

Figure 9.6: Decline curl-up up

Efficient Cardio Exercises

Now we will explore how to select the right types of cardio. As was briefly mentioned in chapter 8, what makes for an efficient cardio exercise is different from strength training. The sole focus of cardio is to get the heart beating and get you breathing more rapidly. According to the American Heart Association, moderate-intensity exercise should increase your heart rate to 50 to 70 percent of your maximal heart rate (MHR).[5] An MHR is the highest level of cardio intensity you should reach while exercising—pushing yourself beyond this intensity level can be unsafe.

To determine your MHR, use this formula: MHR = 208 – (0.7 × Age).[6] Set a moderate-intensity heart-rate target by multiplying your MHR by 0.5 to 0.7. For example,

- A healthy forty-year-old man's MHR is 180 beats per minute (208 – (0.7 × 40) = 180).

- Then 60 percent of this man's MHR is 108 beats per minute (180 × 0.6 = 108).

Any cardio exercise that raises your heart rate to the moderate-intensity range and sustains it is technically effective. A wide range of cardio exercises can accomplish this. Here are a few examples: jogging, biking, jumping jacks, and jumping rope. Note that many substances, over-the-counter medications, and prescription medications (e.g., caffeine, nicotine, antihistamines, and beta blockers) can affect your heart rate and ability to perform and respond to exercise.[7] This means that using your MHR to set exercise heart-rate targets and gauge your exercise intensity won't be the best approach for many people. Alternative methods for gauging exercise intensity will be discussed in chapter 11.

At-Home Cardio Exercises

Now that you understand what makes for an effective cardio exercise, consider which options will work best in your home-gym setting. Cardio exercises that can't be done in your home gym should be immediately disqualified because they'll limit your ability to quickly alternate back and forth between cardio and strength training. For instance, if you're out on a ten-mile bike ride, it would be impossible to quickly stop and execute a set of pull-ups or weighted lunges. This is a problem because the ability to quickly switch between aerobic and anaerobic work can reduce the total amount of cardio exercise that's necessary. This fact has led to a whole branch of training called *interval training*, which will be covered in greater detail in chapter 11.

For now, just know that the ability to do your cardio and strength training all in your home gym is crucial to keeping workouts short. In most cases, doing interval training will disqualify nonstationary exercises, such as swimming, trail running, or mountain biking. You *might* have enough room to jog if you have a large workout room, garage, or unfinished basement.

Most people will need to resort to a stationary form of cardio exercise. A wide variety of options are available; some require special equipment while others do not. For instance, stationary bikes, treadmills, and elliptical machines are common examples of cardio machines. Each of these makes it possible to get a great aerobic workout at home, but they tend to be expensive and take up significant space. Unless you have a physiological problem that requires the use of a machine—such as bad knees—a cardio machine probably isn't necessary. You can do stationary cardio without machines.

Simple Cardio Options

When it comes to selecting cardio exercises to do at home, choosing a simple option is best. This brief section will provide a few basic exercise recommendations, but it's not an exhaustive list. We went into much greater detail on strength-training exercises because designing an exercise program that effectively works all the major muscle groups inherently requires doing many different types of exercises—it's a much more complex task. Selecting a cardio exercise that effectively raises your heart rate to the appropriate level and sustains it can be much more straightforward, so we won't go into as much detail on options and procedures. Remember, this book is not meant to be a technical guide on exercise technique because those resources are widely available and accessible.

The simplest stationary cardio option for most people will be running in place. Though it works different muscles than normal running, running in place is still an effective aerobic exercise. Running in place is exactly what its name implies: you mimic the activity of running but without propelling your body forward. The main difference is that you use your toes and balls of your feet more because you are lifting your knees straight up without any forward motion. To run in place, use your upper body to move your arms back and forth while doing alternating knee raises to about hip height. When doing this relatively quickly, you are basically bouncing from one foot to the other as you alternate knee raises, which mimics the activity of running. To change intensity, change the speed at which you alternate knee raises.[8]

Another good stationary cardio option is jumping jacks. Jumping jacks are an effective aerobic exercise and a great alternative to traditional cardio options like running or biking. They don't require equipment and can be done anywhere. To perform jumping jacks, stand straight up with your arms at your sides. Start by jumping and spreading your feet wider than your hips while simultaneously bringing your arms together above your head. Then jump again, bringing your feet back together while bringing your arms back down to your sides. Continue repeating this process in rhythm for as long as needed. You can adjust the cardio intensity by changing the pace of each jump and hand motion. Note that jumping jacks are a higher impact exercise, so they may not be the best option for people who are pregnant or have knee or ankle problems.[9]

The last at-home stationary exercise that we will explore is jumping rope. Jumping rope can provide a great cardio workout and can be easily performed in most home-gym settings. To do it, buy a jump rope and adjust it to fit your height. All that's required to jump rope is to hold a rope handle in each hand and begin doing revolutions while jumping. Each time the rope swings overhead, be prepared to jump as it descends, which will let it pass beneath your feet and begin the next revolution. It can take some practice to execute properly, but with a little sustained effort, most people can master the basic movement relatively quickly.

An important aspect to focus on when jumping rope is your jump height. When in proper rhythm, you don't need to jump high to allow the rope to pass under your feet. In fact, practiced jumpers usually only come one inch or so off the floor each time they jump. In addition to minimizing jump height, you should also focus on how you land. Land high on your toes (rather than flatfooted or on your heels) to minimize impact. When done properly, jumping rope can be a lower impact cardio exercise than jogging or running. Also, be sure to jump rope on a forgiving surface. A mat or wood floor is preferred over concrete (which is too hard) or carpet (which can make jumping difficult).[10]

Many more viable cardio options can certainly be effective in a home-gym setting, but the three just described are among the simplest and most well-known options. Remember that the goal of cardio exercise is to raise your heart rate to an appropriate level and sustain it; any exercise that can do this and be performed in your home gym can be a good option. Note here that though other forms of cardio that can't be done in a home gym—such as going for an outdoor run or bike ride—may not be ideal for your daily workout routine, you still might enjoy doing them. That is okay. Exercises in the latter category just aren't the most efficient way of meeting your cardio requirements. Think of these types of cardio as an optional supplement to your daily exercise routine if you choose to do them.

Choosing Your Exercises

If you haven't already done so, select the strength-training and cardio exercises that will be the basis of your workout plan. As you make your decisions, remember to keep the following factors in mind: efficiency, safety, your personal capabilities, available space in your home gym, equipment requirements, and budget. Select one exercise for each category:

1. Horizontal push
2. Horizontal pull

3. Vertical push
4. Vertical pull (triceps dominant)
5. Vertical pull (biceps dominant)
6. Hip-dominant pull
7. Quad-dominant push
8. Core exercise
9. Cardio exercise

Table 9.1 shows a variety of different options for each exercise type based on some hypothetical but common home-gym scenarios. While these are by no means the only options, they're practical for most people. Feel free to use them as a guide to help you select exercises. (For more on this, see chapter 10.) If you discover alternative exercises that still align with the principles of high efficiency and low friction, and they work better for your situation, then adopt them. If more efficient and safer exercises are developed in the future, then adopt them. Even if better types of exercises are developed one day (they probably will be), the basic principles for exercise selection presented in this book will stand the test of time.

Choosing Warm-up Exercises

In addition to selecting the exercises that will be used in your workouts, you also need to select warm-up exercises for each compound movement that you'll perform during your workouts. Using bodyweight or resistance band exercises for your warm-up routine is often best. The main reason for this is that warm-ups are meant only to prepare the specific body parts that you're about to exercise for movement, so overburdening muscles with too much resistance at this stage isn't necessary. When done correctly, a proper warm-up can prepare the nervous system for more challenging loads, enhance balance and coordination, and may help reduce the risk of injury.[11]

Table 9.1

Suggested Exercises

Exercise type	Minimal equipment and space	Moderate equipment and space	Maximum equipment and space
1. Horizontal push	Push-ups or resistance band chest press	Barbell or dumbbell bench press	Bench press machine
2. Horizontal pull	Resistance band rows	One-arm dumbbell rows	Rowing machine
3. Vertical push	Pike press or resistance band shoulder press	Seated shoulder press	Shoulder press machine
4. Vertical pull (triceps dominant)	Pull-ups or resistance band pull-downs	Pull-ups or resistance band pull-downs	Machine pull-downs, palms down
5. Vertical pull (biceps dominant)	Chin-ups or resistance band pull-downs	Chin-ups or resistance band pull-downs	Machine pull-downs, palms up
6. Hip-dominant exercise	Resistance band dead lifts	Dead lift or rack pulls	Weighted back extensions
7. Quad-dominant exercise	Resistance band or body-weight squats	Dumbbell lunges	Leg press machine
8. Core exercise	Abdominal crunches	Decline bench curl-ups	Ab crunch machine
9. Cardio exercise	Run in place or jumping jacks	Jump rope	Stationary bike, treadmill, or elliptical machine

Using body-weight or resistance-band exercises helps reduce friction by allowing you to warm up quickly before your workout; this approach eliminates the need to change weights or adjust resistance on equipment that you're about to use. For instance, warming up for bench presses by doing push-ups or resistance band presses can allow you to effectively warm up your chest and arms without having to stop and increase weights on your bench press before starting your workout. If you warm up with the same exercises and equipment that you're about to use, you will have to stop and adjust equipment before starting your workout because your warm-ups will require using less weight or resistance. This is a phenomenon called equipment overlap (which is discussed further in chapter 10). To select appropriate warm-up exercises, refer to the body-weight and resistance band exercises discussed in chapter 8.

Conclusion

In this chapter, you learned about additional types of exercises—beyond the six essential compound movements—that should be included in your low-friction program. You now know that most isolation (single-joint) exercises aren't required for basic muscle strengthening and development and that they can significantly increase the length of workouts. You've learned that ab exercises should be included in your program because they can strengthen midsection muscles, which can help prevent injury by stabilizing the spine. You've also learned that ideal cardio exercises for a low-friction routine should be able to be performed inside your home gym and should be capable of raising your heart rate and sustaining it at an appropriate level. Finally, you learned how to select appropriate warm-up exercises to get each muscle group efficiently prepared for more challenging movement. By learning about these additional types of exercises, you've gained the fundamental knowledge required to select all the exercises that will be the basis of your personalized low-friction workout routine.

CHAPTER 10

Starting to Design Your Program

ONCE YOU'VE SELECTED THE INDIVIDUAL exercises that will be included in your workout program, you're ready to begin structuring the program itself. To do so, develop a series of different twenty-minute daily workouts that consistently utilize all the exercises you've selected. This will require you to grasp and consider all the exercise factors discussed in this chapter and the next one. Below is a list of the key considerations for program development that will be covered in this chapter:

- Figuring out how to group the right exercises together for individual daily workouts
- Doing your different daily workouts in the right order over time
- Allowing adequate recovery time between workouts
- Deciding which strength exercises will compose your three different workouts
- Determining how many sets of repetitions you will do for each exercise
- Selecting the right number of individual repetitions to do within each set

- Determining the right amount of weight or resistance for strength-training exercises

These key factors will help you get started on designing your workout program.

Grouping the Right Exercises

First, we'll cover how to divide up your strength exercises into separate daily workouts. Since your individual workouts will only last twenty minutes, each one should include only two to three of these exercises—plus your cardio exercise. Each workout should include different strength exercises. This means that you shouldn't use the same exercise in multiple daily workouts. For instance, you wouldn't include bench presses in your workouts over two consecutive days.

To make your exercise sessions as efficient as possible, avoid grouping any exercises into the same workout that have overlapping equipment needs. In other words, you shouldn't be doing exercises that require using the same weights, dumbbells, or bar on the same day. Avoiding equipment overlap eliminates the need to stop during a workout to move or adjust equipment, which can significantly decrease the time required for an exercise session. For instance, putting bench press and dead lift into the same session would be a mistake because they both require using the barbell (weight bar). You'd have to stop to change weights and move the bar *during* this workout, which would create unnecessary friction.

Tables 10.1, 10.2, and 10.3 show multiple examples of how you could group various exercises to minimize transition time. Notice that some of the daily workout groupings vary between scenarios depending on the specific exercises chosen and the equipment needed.

Table 10.1

Home-Gym Scenario: Moderate Equipment and Space

Workout	Exercise type	Exercise	Equipment required
Daily workout 1	Horizontal push	Barbell bench press	Bench and barbell set
	Vertical push	Seated shoulder press	Bench and dumbbells
	Stationary cardio exercise	Jump rope	Jump rope
Daily workout 2	Vertical pull (triceps dominant)	Pull-ups or resistance band pull-downs	Pull-up bar or resistance bands
	Vertical pull (biceps dominant)	Chin-ups or resistance band pull-downs	Pull-up bar or resistance bands
	Horizontal pull	One-arm dumbbell rows	Bench and dumbbells
	Stationary cardio exercise	Jump rope	Jump rope
Daily workout 3	Hip-dominant exercise	Dead lift or rack pulls	Weighted barbell
	Quad-dominant exercise	Dumbbell lunges	Dumbbells
	Core exercise	Abdominal crunch	Dumbbell or single weight plate
	Stationary cardio exercise	Jump rope	Jump rope

Table 10.2

Home-Gym Scenario: Maximum Equipment and Space

WORKOUT	EXERCISE TYPE	EXERCISE	EQUIPMENT REQUIRED
Daily workout 1	Horizontal push	Chest press	Bench press machine
	Horizontal pull	Seated rows	Rowing machine
	Stationary cardio exercise	Elliptical machine	Elliptical machine
Daily workout 2	Vertical push	Shoulder press	Shoulder press machine
	Vertical pull (biceps dominant)	Machine pull-downs, palms up	Pull-down machine
	Hip-dominant exercise	Weighted back extensions	Hyperextension bench and dumbbells
	Stationary cardio exercise	Elliptical machine	Elliptical machine
Daily workout 3	Vertical pull (triceps dominant)	Machine pull-downs, palms downs	Pull-down machine
	Quad-dominant exercise	Leg press	Leg press machine
	Stationary cardio exercise	Elliptical machine	Elliptical machine
	Core exercise	Abdominal crunch	Ab crunch machine

Table 10.3
Home-Gym Scenario: Minimal Equipment and Space

Workout	Exercise type	Exercise	Equipment required
Daily workout 1	Horizontal push	Push-ups or resistance band chest press	Resistance bands
	Vertical push	Pike press or resistance band shoulder press	Resistance bands
	Stationary cardio exercise	Jumping jacks or run in place	none
Daily workout 2	Horizontal pull	Resistance band rows	Resistance bands
	Vertical pull (triceps dominant)	Pull-ups or resistance band pull-downs	Pull-up bar or resistance bands
	Vertical pull (biceps dominant)	Chin-ups or resistance band pull-downs	Pull-up bar or resistance bands
	Stationary cardio exercise	Jumping jacks or run in place	none
Daily workout 3	Hip-dominant exercise	Resistance band dead lifts	Resistance bands
	Quad-dominant exercise	Resistance band or body-weight squats	Resistance bands
	Stationary cardio exercise	Jumping jacks or run in place	none
	Core exercise	Abdominal Crunch	none

First, we'll examine the moderate-equipment-and-space scenario in table 10.1 because it's the most common situation. Notice that the exercises selected for each daily workout have no overlapping equipment needs. For example, daily workout 1 requires an exercise bench and barbell set for bench presses and the exercise bench and dumbbells for seated shoulder presses. This grouping works well because you can quickly transition from bench presses to shoulder presses without having to unload the barbell and move weights. Notice the same dynamic in daily workout 2, which pairs a triceps-dominant vertical pull, biceps-dominant vertical pull, and horizontal pull exercise. Both types of vertical pull utilize body weight and possibly one weighted dumbbell for those that need an additional challenge. The other dumbbell can be set to a different weight and used for one-arm dumbbell rows. Here again, you'd waste no time switching between these exercises. This friction-free dynamic is also seen in the daily workout 3 grouping. Dead lifts use a weighted barbell, lunges use weighted dumbbells, and crunches are done with just body weight or while holding a single weight plate, so this workout is also designed for quick transitions between exercises.

Next, let's examine the maximum-equipment-and-space scenario. If you're fortunate enough to have lots of space for a home gym and the funds for several workout machines, you'll enjoy a bit more flexibility in your plan. You'll still need to be strategic in how you group your exercises to avoid equipment overlap. Notice in the example plan that none of the exercises within a single workout require using the same equipment for more than one exercise. For instance, in daily workout number one, you would use a chest press machine, a seated rowing machine, and an elliptical machine. You could easily switch exercises within this grouping without stopping to move or adjust equipment.

Finally, we'll explore the minimal-equipment-and-space scenario. The benefit of this approach is that it provides ultimate flexibility in how daily workouts can be structured. You can easily transition between any of the exercises regardless of how they're organized because no weights, barbells, or other equipment need to be adjusted. Notice the way the various exercises have been grouped: upper-body pushing exercises on day one, upper-body pulling exercises on day two, and lower-body and core exercises on day three. While this scheme works, these exercises could be paired into virtually any combination without creating equipment overlap problems.

While the minimal-equipment approach does make it easier to devise twenty-minute workouts, this strategy can be limiting in the long run. The main problem is with body-weight exercises like push-ups and body-weight squats. While they are fantastic for beginners and great options when you're traveling, you'll eventually need exercises that are more adequately challenging. At some point you'll require more strength-training resistance to continue maintaining and developing your muscles. To get adequate strength training, everyone should eventually transition to free weights or exercise machines. If this isn't possible, you can get some great heavy-duty resistance band sets that provide appropriate levels of resistance.

Scheduling Your Workouts over Time

Since you'll only be doing two to three of your strength exercises during each daily session, you should have a total of three different workouts. You should consistently cycle through these workouts in consecutive order over time, which means continually repeating the following pattern:

Day 1: Do workout 1.
Day 2: Do workout 2.
Day 3: Do workout 3.
Day 4: Do workout 1.

With this approach, you'll do the same series of workouts, in the same order repetitively for months, years, and hopefully even decades. Table 10.4 shows an example of what your progression of daily exercises looks like over the course of one month.

You shouldn't change your workout pattern unless you have a legitimate reason to do so. Here are a few examples of circumstances that might warrant a change to your workout pattern:

- You need to change one of your strength exercises or pieces of equipment.
- You'll be traveling or away from your home gym for an extended period.
- You sustain an injury that requires you to stop doing a specific type of exercise.

Adjusting for Recovery Time

A big benefit of dividing up your strength exercises into a three-day rotation is that it allows individual muscles to get the recovery time they need because you'll work different muscle groups from workout to workout, never doing the same strength exercises on consecutive days. Following a three-day rotation results in working each muscle group two to three times per week, which aligns with the American College of Sports Medicine fitness guidelines.[1] While a three-workout plan is the general recommendation, different people need various amounts of time for recovery. Factors such as age, training experience, exercise volume, and sleep patterns can affect your recovery requirements.

If after implementing your three-day plan you find that you need more recovery time, you can change to a four- or five-day plan. Before doing so, consider each of the following:

Table 10.4

Example of Daily Workout Progression

Week 1	Daily Workout	Week 2	Daily Workout	Week 3	Daily Workout	Week 4	Daily Workout	Week 5	Daily Workout
1/1	Workout 1	1/8	Workout 2	1/15	Workout 3	1/22	Workout 1	1/29	Workout 2
1/2	Workout 2	1/9	Workout 3	1/16	Workout 1	1/23	Workout 2	1/30	Workout 3
1/3	Workout 3	1/10	Workout 1	1/17	Workout 2	1/24	Workout 3	1/31	Workout 1
1/4	Workout 1	1/11	Workout 2	1/18	Workout 3	1/25	Workout 1		
1/5	Workout 2	1/12	Workout 3	1/19	Workout 1	1/26	Workout 2		
1/6	Workout 3	1/13	Workout 1	1/20	Workout 2	1/27	Workout 3		
1/7	Workout 1	1/14	Workout 2	1/21	Workout 3	1/28	Workout 1		

Soreness—Anyone not used to regular exercise is going to be sore in the beginning, so soreness isn't necessarily a legitimate reason to extend recovery time. Being so sore that you can't move is one thing, but just mild soreness often means that you had a good workout. Give your body a few weeks to get used to regular training; in most cases you will easily adjust to mild soreness.

Sleep—If you're consistently going four or five days without fully recovering from workouts, you may not be getting enough sleep. Getting enough sleep is one of the most efficient ways to ensure you'll get optimal recovery—many people just aren't getting enough. Be sure that you're getting the recommended seven to nine hours per night to maximize recovery.[2]

Intensity—If you can't recover in three days, you may be pushing yourself too hard. Training should be challenging but not grueling. Sometimes, slightly reducing cardio intensity and resistance levels can help make recovery easier.

If none of these considerations help you, then you can build some extra recovery time into your plan. To do so, just add extra cardio-only workout days to your plan as needed. For instance, if you need an extra day to fully recover, you would just add a fourth day of cardio-only to your exercise rotation. Again, a three-day plan is generally adequate for most people.

Finalizing Your Strength-Training Splits

After learning all the relevant considerations, you're now ready to decide how to split up your strength exercises into your three daily workouts. This will probably take you about thirty minutes to one hour, but once the plan is complete, you'll be able to follow it for many years to come. Remember to keep exercise transition time in mind as you do this—this will ensure that your workouts are as efficient as possible. Going through this planning process *prior* to purchasing any weights or equipment is helpful because as you plan, you may realize that certain gear might work better within your system or space than other options.

Determining the Right Number of Sets

The next step is to determine the number of sets you'll do of each strength exercise during each workout. Doing three sets of each strength exercise is ideal because it allows for strength building and muscle development while keeping workouts short. Many trainers advocate doing as many as five or six sets per exercise, but this generally isn't necessary. If you want to go beyond three sets, you can, but keep long-term sustainability in mind. Doing more than three sets of each exercise will make workouts longer. If you do ever need to increase your rep volume to continue making progress, an alternative strategy to increasing sets is doing slower reps. This approach lengthens the amount of time that your muscles are under tension without having to add sets to your workout. In general, three sets of each exercise should be enough to adequately work the major muscle groups.

You might be wondering, Why do I need to break up my strength-training reps into multiple sets? Can't I just bang out all my reps for each strength exercise in one large set? The answer is no. To adequately work your muscles, do reps with an amount of weight or resistance that can be sustained for only about thirty to sixty seconds. The number of reps you do during these short periods are considered a set. Due to the short amount of time that your muscles can bear to be under tension, you won't be able to complete an adequate number of reps in a single set. To complete enough total reps during each workout, perform multiple sets with recovery time taken in between.

Setting Rep Volume and Stimulating Muscle Growth

Next, decide how many individual reps of each exercise to do within a set. The three most common rep quantity ranges are shown in table 10.5.

High-rep training is fantastic for building muscular endurance, which is why it's often used in sports training—athletes need this type of strength training to prevent muscle fatigue during competition. The problem with it as a primary solution is that it requires exercising with relatively low amounts of resistance.[3] While this method can be effective at helping you build and develop muscle mass, it's less effective at helping increase overall strength. While gaining strength should not be your primary goal, it shouldn't be neglected because it can impact your mobility, especially later in life.

Low-rep training requires exercising with resistance that's at or near your one-rep maximum (i.e., the amount of resistance with which you can complete only one full repetition). This type of training delivers the best results when it comes to purely building strength, and this makes it the method of choice for sports where power is king—such

Table 10.5
Ranges of Rep Volume

TYPE OF TRAINING	REP VOLUME PER SET
High rep	15 or more
Moderate rep	8–12
Low rep	5 or fewer

Source: Michael Berg and Brad Schoenfeld, "How Many Reps Will Build the Most Muscle?" Men's Journal, May 22, 2020, https://www.mensjournal.com /health-fitness/rep-range-builds-most-muscle/.

as powerlifting. The downside of low-rep training is that though it can stimulate some muscle growth, it's not the optimal means of doing so. This is the case because your muscles are under tension for less time during the shorter sets with fewer reps—usually fifteen seconds or less. This isn't a problem for powerlifters because they prefer to gain strength while building as little additional mass as possible. Doing low reps is a problem if you care about muscle mass since optimal muscle growth is induced when muscles are under tension for thirty to sixty seconds. When muscles are kept under adequate tension for longer, they are exhausted of energy *and* put under mechanical stress—which optimizes muscle growth.[4]

If your primary goal is to improve your body composition while also building some strength, then moderate-rep training is generally the best option. Moderate-rep training is optimal because it puts muscles under significant tension for the ideal thirty- to sixty-second time frame. To achieve this, you should aim to do three sets of eight to twelve reps with challenging resistance for each strength exercise. In most cases, this will allow you to build muscle and strength faster than a low- or high-rep approach.

At this point you're probably wondering whether there's ever a reason to do high-rep or low-rep sets. The answer is yes, but only in certain cases:

- You're trying to increase strength but have hit a plateau that you can't break through with sets of eight to twelve.
- You're trying to increase muscle mass, and doing sets of eight to twelve has stopped being effective.

First, we'll address the strength plateau. An important component of strength training is gradually increasing the amount of resistance you exercise with. Doing this is necessary to keep exercises adequately challenging for your muscles. As you progress, you'll sometimes hit strength plateaus that are difficult to break through. When this occurs, temporarily changing up your rep strategy can be helpful for breaking through the plateau. For instance, if your strength at a certain exercise won't increase, you can try a heavier low-rep or a lighter high-rep routine for about a month or so. These types of temporary changes in volume and resistance have shown to be effective at increasing strength.[5] After this period, you would return to doing moderate-rep sets to see whether you're able to resume making strength increases.

Next, we'll address the halt in your progress of developing muscle mass. If you're attempting to build more muscle and consistently doing sets of eight to twelve reps has ceased to be effective, a temporary change in rep strategy can help. Before you make a change, you should verify that you're eating right and getting adequate rest and recovery because these factors are often the problem. Once you've ruled out diet, rest, and recovery, making a temporary change to your rep strategy is advisable. As with the strength-plateau scenario, you can try a heavier low-rep or a lighter high-rep routine for a month or so before returning to your normal eight- to twelve-rep approach. In studies, such changes in resistance and rep volume have shown to increase muscle development.[6]

Changing your rep strategy is necessary only when you're trying to increase strength or muscle mass and moderate-rep training stops being effective. This means that there's no reason to change if

- The moderate-rep approach is working for you, which will often be the case—especially if you haven't been strength training for many years.
- You're successfully maintaining your strength and muscle mass and have no need or interest in increasing them further.

While temporarily cycling through other rep ranges can be helpful in certain situations, your primary strategy should be doing moderate-rep sets with challenging levels of resistance.

Also note that changing your rep volume is not the only way to break through strength plateaus or stimulate muscle growth. The fundamental requirement for either is to make a change to the way you're exercising that forces your body to adapt to new conditions. As was previously mentioned, changing the amount of time that muscles are under tension by slowing down your repetitions is another great way to force muscle adaptation. For instance, people who normally execute individual repetitions in two to four seconds could slow down their movement so their reps take four to six seconds.

Another effective way of encouraging adaptation is to make a slight variation to the way you perform a strength exercise—such as changing a hand grip or stance. For instance, people struggling to gain strength on the bench press might try temporarily widening or narrowing their grip by an inch or two.

The broad point is you can change up an exercise when necessary in different ways and doing so doesn't have to be complicated. Your overarching rep strategy for strength training should be as follows: Default to doing eight to twelve reps with challenging resistance unless this approach stops being effective at making progress toward your strength or development goals. If a change is needed to further progress, try temporarily cycling to high- or low-rep sets, changing rep speed, or changing hand grips or stances.

Calibrating Resistance for Strength Training

Now that you understand the benefits of doing three sets of eight to twelve repetitions for each strength exercise, you'll need to learn to determine how much weight or resistance to use. The general rule is to use an amount of resistance at which you can complete each set, but you should be near muscle failure on the final rep of each set. Ideally, failure would occur if you attempted one additional rep beyond your rep target. For example, a man is doing a seated shoulder press, and his goal is to do three sets of ten repetitions with thirty-pound dumbbells. The weight is challenging, but he's able to complete ten reps for each set. If he were to attempt an eleventh rep, his muscles would fail, and he wouldn't be able to complete the final repetition.

To select an appropriate amount of resistance for each of your exercises, do some experimenting. This requires devoting roughly an hour (or multiple shorter sessions) to calibrating your resistance levels for each strength exercise. This calibration session will take longer than a standard workout, but you'll need to do it only once to gauge your baseline strength levels.

If you have no idea how much resistance to start with, begin by attempting eight to twelve reps of each exercise with a low amount of weight. Try five to ten pounds for dumbbell exercises and ten to twenty pounds for barbell exercises. If using machines or other non-free-weight resistance equipment, start with one of the lowest resistance settings. If you have some strength-training experience, you may already have a rough idea of what the right resistance amounts are. In this situation, start calibrating with an amount of resistance nearer to your known capabilities.

Regardless of where you begin calibrating, the first step is to do eight to twelve repetitions of each strength exercise with those initial amounts of weight. After completing the first round of sets, you'll then need to consider their difficulty and decide whether you're capable of increasing the resistance. If so, add five to ten pounds of resistance to each exercise and then attempt a second round of sets. Just ensure that you take three to five minutes to rest between sets. Continue this process of increasing resistance and completing sets until you find resistance levels that are appropriately challenging. Again, at the ideal resistance level, your last rep should be difficult to complete.

Some people will be capable of increasing resistance between sets by more than five to ten pounds at a time. Doing so is fine if you're able, just keep in mind that increasing resistance in smaller increments is advisable for avoiding injury. After completing this calibration process, you'll know the baseline levels of resistance that you should begin working out with.

Conclusion

In this chapter, you began learning about how to structure your exercise program by developing a repeating series of twenty-minute daily workouts. You now know how to reduce friction by grouping the right strength exercises into three different workouts based on equipment and space, avoid equipment overlap, and avoid overtraining by doing your daily exercises in the right order over time. You've learned that the ideal low-friction twenty-minute workout includes three sets of each exercise and doing eight to twelve repetitions within each set. You also learned why working out with a challenging level of resistance that brings you near failure on your final rep of each set is important and how to appropriately calibrate the right weight and resistance levels to use for each exercise. By learning about these important factors, you've made significant progress toward building the fundamental knowledge base required to create an effective low-friction workout routine.

CHAPTER 11

Finalizing Your Workout Program

TO HELP YOU FINALIZE THE design of your workout program let's explore more considerations for building effective twenty-minute daily workouts:

- The value of and methods for tracking your exercise performance
- When to increase weight or resistance for strength-training exercises
- How long to rest between sets
- How to integrate cardio into your workouts
- The value of twenty-minute workouts—versus shorter workouts
- How to set your target heart rate for cardio
- Ways to gauge your heart rate during workouts
- How to get started tomorrow

Documenting Strength Gains and Performance

Once you've identified the baseline resistance levels for your workouts, document them. This documentation process shouldn't be a one-time occurrence; it should happen after each daily exercise session. This is important because the amounts of resistance you exercise with will change over time, and it'll be nearly impossible to remember them all. If you can't remember how much weight or resistance to use for your exercises, then there will be a lot more friction when you're prepping your equipment. When you have a performance log, this is not a problem. You just consult the log and see exactly how much weight to use.

The other major benefit of regular performance documentation is that it forces you to notice the strength gains you've made. Even if you don't care about strength, getting stronger is a good indication that you're *at least* preventing muscle loss—if not developing some additional muscle mass. Seeing the performance improvements you've made over time in your log is motivating because they affirm that your exercise program is working.

For example, in a previous workout Vanessa did ten reps of dumbbell lunges in her first two sets but could complete only eight reps on the third set. On her next lunge day, she does ten reps in the first two sets and can now complete ten reps on her third set. In this scenario, Vanessa's body has recovered and responded positively to her previous workout. Getting these regular affirmations of progress can be helpful because progress isn't always clear at the daily level from body-composition metrics. As you've learned, taking weekly or monthly averages from body weight, body fat, and FFMI is sometimes necessary to recognize real progress. People tend to get disheartened when the scale or body fat calipers don't show more immediate evidence of improvement on a given day. When this happens, recognizing and documenting that you have made a performance improvement is a powerful reminder that your system is working.

You can use any one of many methods to keep a record of exercise performance. You can create a pen-and-paper log in a journal or notebook, use a digital spreadsheet, or utilize a note-taking app on a smart phone or other mobile device. Any of these can be effective if it keeps track of the following:

- The exercises done during each workout
- How much weight or resistance was used for each exercise and workout
- How many sets and repetitions were performed for each exercise and workout

After completing every workout, take a minute or two to open your log and update it with the latest performance data. If you can establish and maintain this practice, you will greatly increase your chances of making exercise a lifelong habit.

Learning When to Increase Strength-Training Resistance

To make progress with your new exercise program, you'll need to know when and by how much to increase strength-training resistance over time. First, recognize that everyone doesn't gain strength at the same pace. Age, sex, genetics, and many other factors all impact how quickly you develop strength. The best way to determine when to increase the resistance on a given exercise is to consider how easily you're able to complete the final repetitions in each set. If you're capable of doing additional reps in your last set—beyond what's planned—without taking a break, then you should increase weight or resistance. For instance, if you're doing three sets of ten reps on a bench press and you're capable of completing eleven reps on the last set, then you should increase the weight next time you do bench presses.

Determining how much to increase resistance requires taking many factors into account. The type of exercise, the amount of time you've been training, and your age, sex, and genetics all play a role. A good general rule is to increase the resistance by 5 to 10 percent once you're able to complete all your reps with proper technique without experiencing muscle failure.[1] Recognize that you may need to do some individual calibrating to get your resistance increases right. Also, remember that you will probably make large strength gains during the first few months if you're new to strength training. But your capacity for quickly building strength will taper off as you build experience.

After many years of consistent training, you may reach a stage at which you're making strength gains of only one pound or less at a time. When you reach this advanced stage, having a set of ultralight weights to help you continue increasing resistance in small increments is beneficial. The best tools for this are called fractional weight plates, which weigh one pound or less. You can buy them individually or in sets of various sizes. For those using resistance bands, you can also buy very low-tension bands to incrementally add resistance. While counterintuitive, consistently adding fractional amounts of resistance to your exercises can compound into significant increases over time.

Resting between Sets

The final component of building a proper strength-training program is incorporating adequate recovery periods between each set in your workout. The three basic types of rest period are: short, medium, and long (see table 11.1).

Short rest periods are great for high-rep strength training but generally aren't used for moderate- or low-rep training. The main problem with short rests is that they don't allow most people's muscles enough time to sufficiently recover from lifting a challenging weight.[2]

Long rest periods give you enough time to recover strength more fully, which enables you to exercise with more resistance. They are

Table 11.1

Types of Recovery between Sets

RECOVERY TYPE	REST PERIOD	BENEFIT
Short	30 seconds or less	Muscular endurance
Medium	30–90 seconds	Muscular growth
Long	2–5 minutes	Strength and power

Source: G. Gregory Haff and N. Travis Triplett, *Essentials of Strength Training and Conditioning,* 4th ed. (Illinois: Human Kinetics, 2016), 465.

great for purely building strength but are less effective when it comes to maximizing muscle growth. When you take longer rests, pushing your muscles to maximum exhaustion is harder because they have too much time to recover.[3] The other drawback of long rest periods is that they dramatically increase the length of workouts. For instance, if you're taking five-minute breaks between sets and your workout includes two exercises, you'll spend twenty-five minutes just on recovery. Taking this much time to rest is a problem if your aim is to keep workouts short.

To maximize muscle development, you want to make a *partial recovery* between sets. This means resting just enough to allow you to complete the next set—not enough to fully recover. Medium (thirty to ninety second) rest periods are ideal for this.[4] Factors such as your age and level of fitness may require you to take longer rests between sets, at least until your stamina is built up more. If you consistently find that medium rest periods aren't enough recovery to complete your next set, then you're probably using too much weight or resistance. If you experience this, reduce the resistance for your exercises until a medium rest period provides enough recovery.

Incorporating Cardio

Your workouts should also have cardio exercise efficiently incorporated into them. The best way to keep the amount of daily time you spend exercising to twenty minutes is to use a method called interval training. Interval training requires alternating between short bursts of intense exercise and less intense periods of exercise.[5] A simple example of interval training would be alternating between short fifteen- to thirty-second bursts of hard running and thirty to ninety seconds of light jogging. The short intense bursts of activity increase your average heart rate close to its maximum. The periods of less intense exercise allow the heart rate to drop but prevent it from dropping too low. Over the course of a twenty-minute workout, this pattern results in a moderately high average heart rate, which helps effectively meet the basic cardio exercise intensity and duration requirements for most people healthy enough to exercise.

Interval training is extremely efficient because it allows you to combine strength training and cardio into one workout session and get the benefits of both.[6] The key to this is using strength exercises as your short intense bursts. When you do eight to twelve reps of a strength exercise with challenging resistance, your heart rate comes close to its maximal rate. In traditional strength-training programs, most people just sit or stand still during their rest periods, which allows their heart rate to fall to its normal resting rate. With interval training, you can take advantage of the elevated heart rate that strength exercises cause by not allowing your heart rate to drop back down to its resting rate after completing a set. To achieve this, you need to do some type of moderately paced cardio activity in between the intense strength-training sets. For instance, after completing ten repetitions of bench press, you could jog in place or jump rope for thirty to ninety seconds while recovering—instead of just sitting or standing.

Afterward, you'd go right into another set on the bench press. Doing this keeps your average heart rate in the cardio range for your entire exercise session, meaning that the whole workout—even the strength training—counts as cardio.

By building many different exercises into one interval-training program (sometimes called circuit training), you turn standard strength workouts into anaerobic *and* aerobic workouts. This means you don't need to spend additional time doing cardio exercise because you get what you need out of one short workout. With this approach, you meet all the basic exercise requirements in much less time, which greatly increases the chances of making exercise a sustainable habit.

Upon learning about interval training, the most common question is, Will I be able to adequately recover from strength exercises if I'm doing cardio in between sets? The answer is yes! The beauty of interval training is that it takes advantage of the difference between anaerobic and aerobic work. While doing bouts of cardio, the lactic acid "burn" caused by a strength exercise will die down, which will prepare you for more strength training sets (this is sometimes called active recovery).[7] Table 11.2 gives an example of what a twenty-minute interval-training workout that includes strength-training exercises looks like.

Making Your Workouts Last Twenty Minutes

At this point, many people wonder, What if I get through all my strength-training exercises in less than twenty minutes? Can I cut my exercise session short? You can definitely finish in less than twenty minutes—this often happens when you take less than one-minute recovery periods between sets. But cutting the workout short when this happens isn't advisable because doing so results in a lessened cardio benefit. If you finish your strength exercises in under twenty minutes, try one or more of these suggestions:

Table 11.2

Example of Interval Training Workout

Exercise	Intensity	Minutes
Abdominal crunch	High	1:00
Cardio	Moderate	1:00
Abdominal crunch	High	1:00
Cardio	Moderate	1:00
Abdominal crunch	High	1:00
Cardio	Moderate	1:00
Dead lift	High	1:00
Cardio	Moderate	1:00
Dead lift	High	1:00
Cardio	Moderate	1:00
Dead lift	High	1:00
Cardio	Moderate	1:00
Dumbbell lunges (both legs)	High	2:00
Cardio	Moderate	1:00
Dumbbell lunges (both legs)	High	2:00
Cardio	Moderate	1:00
Dumbbell lunges (both legs)	High	2:00
Total workout time:		20:00

- You can do your moderately paced cardio exercise for the remainder of the workout until you hit the twenty-minute mark.
- You can keep doing interval training by doing thirty second bouts of harder cardio for your intense sets (in place of strength-training sets). You'd also still do thirty to ninety seconds of moderate cardio during your recovery periods.
- You can keep doing interval training by completing extra strength-training sets with moderate cardio during the rest periods. For instance, you could do a fourth or fifth set of dead lifts or lunges.
- You can keep doing interval training by adding some isolation exercises (such as biceps curls or triceps extensions) to your daily routine.

Note that the third and fourth options can make your workout significantly more difficult, so think carefully about what'll be most sustainable for you long term. Ultimately, how you choose to utilize any remaining time in your workout to reach the twenty-minute mark is a matter of personal preference. Spend any extra time on exercises that prevent your average heart rate from falling too low.

Setting Your Target Heart Rate

By doing 20 minutes of interval training per day, you'll be doing 140 minutes of cardio exercise per week. At 140 minutes, the interval-style workouts will exceed the 150 minutes of moderate-intensity exercise recommended by the CDC because of the brief bouts of strength training included in the workouts. Remember that your strength-training sets count as intense exercise, and every minute of intense exercise counts as 2 minutes of moderate-intensity exercise.[8]

Assume that each strength-training set takes 1 minute to complete. With six to nine total sets in each session, you'll spend 6–9 minutes of every workout doing intense exercise—which equates to 12–18 minutes of moderate cardio. This means that each 20-minute interval workout is equivalent to 26–29 minutes of moderate exercise, thus your daily workouts will count as 182–203 minutes of moderate exercise weekly.

The CDC and American Heart Association consider a heart rate between 50 and 70 percent of your MHR moderate intensity, so make this your target range for cardio. To determine your target heart rate, calculate your MHR. As was noted in chapter 9, MHR can be calculated with this formula: MHR = 208 − (0.7 × Age). Certain factors, such as having diabetes, being at risk for heart disease, being a man over the age of forty-five, being a woman over the age of fifty-five, or taking certain types of medication—such as blood pressure medication—can all further decrease your MHR. If any of these risk factors apply to you, disclosing your plans to engage in vigorous exercise to your doctor before getting started is advisable. Note that studies have shown interval-training programs to be well tolerated by most people, even those with heart conditions.[9]

Once you've determined your MHR, you need to calculate what your heart rate would be in the 50 to 70 percent range. For example, a man's target heart rate is 60 percent of his MHR. To make the calculation we would multiply his MHR by his target percentage, which is 0.6. In this case the man's target heart rate would be 108 beats per minute (180 × 0.6 = 108). Your goal while doing bouts of moderate cardio during workouts should be to bring your heart rate near your target—but remember that your heart rate will spike higher at intervals due to your strength-training sets. The result will be 140 minutes of weekly exercise that exceeds the 150-minute minimum.[10]

Gauging Your Heart Rate

After determining what your average target heart rate should be, decide how you'll gauge your heart rate during workouts. The most accurate method is to use some type of personal heart-rate monitor. Many types exist and they vary widely in price and functionality, but nearly all of them provide the two essential functions:

- Displaying your actual heart rate during exercise
- Calculating your average heart rate per workout session

The first function allows you to gauge your real-time heart rate at any point during exercise. The second provides your average heart rate for a workout, which you need to determine whether your cardio intensity is adequate. While you can certainly spend a significant amount of money on a fancy heart-rate monitor, you can generally find an affordable option that's effective. At the time of this writing you can buy a capable heart-rate monitor for less than $30.

While heart-rate monitors are effective, you can also gauge cardio intensity based on how you *feel* during exercise. While taking this approach isn't directly quantifiable, doing so is, in many ways, a better method for determining when you should or shouldn't increase intensity. The recommended intensity level for cardio is moderate, which is any heart rate that falls between 50 and 70 percent of your MHR. According to the Mayo Clinic, moderate-intensity exercise should feel somewhat hard and should cause you the following responses: quickened breath, but not breathless, and a light sweat. (For example, you could carry on a conversation but couldn't sing.)[11]

Conversely, vigorous-intensity exercise has the following effects: deep and rapid breathing and a quick moderate to heavy sweat. (For example, you could only speak a few words without stopping to catch your breath.) A heart rate that falls between 70 and 85 percent of your MHR is considered vigorous.[12] While moderate-intensity exercise is the general recommendation, you could also do vigorous exercise if you are healthy enough to do so. However, doing so on an everyday basis generally isn't sustainable for most people.

You can get surprisingly good at determining how hard your heart is working by watching for these qualitative indicators during exercise. While gauging intensity based on these criteria won't reveal your average heart rate, this method is the simplest option for most people. Is this approach as accurate as a heart-rate monitor? No, but relying on qualitative indicators is accurate enough for general health and fitness in most cases. If you're especially interested in being exact, use a heart-rate monitor, but for most people, the additional effort won't be worth the payoff. Also remember (as was mentioned in chapter 9) that many over-the-counter and prescription medications can affect your heart rate and exercise performance, which can render heart-rate monitors and targets inaccurate and ineffective. If you take any medications or substances that affect your heart rate, gauging intensity based on feeling and bodily responses (such as perceived exertion, pace of breath, and amount of sweat) is usually preferable. If you're unsure which medications or substances could affect your heart rate and exercise performance, you should discuss this with your doctor.

Manipulating Heart Rate

Now that you know how to gauge your heart rate, you can then learn how to manipulate it by changing exercise intensity. With interval training, the most effective way of raising or lowering your average heart rate is by adjusting the intensity of the cardio exercise you do. When starting out, you'll probably need to go through a few workout sessions to determine how hard to push yourself. If your first few workouts are difficult and you think you're pushing beyond moderate intensity, then lessen the intensity of your cardio in the next workout. Likewise, if your first few workouts feel too easy and you think they were below moderate intensity, then increase your cardio intensity in the next workout.

Regardless of whether you're gauging intensity based on feeling or by using a heart-rate monitor, it will take you a bit of time to find your intensity sweet spot. Once you get familiar with where your sweet spot is, reaching and maintaining it will quickly become second nature. Reaching the right intensity level and general heart-rate zone is much more important than hitting an exact target.

Warm-Ups and Cool-Downs

You might be curious about whether warm-up and cool-down periods should be a part of your daily exercise routines. As was mentioned in chapter 9, the purpose of warming up before a workout is to prepare the body for more demanding movements, increase balance and coordination, and help decrease the risk of injury. Cooling down is a postworkout activity (such as stretching) that's used to return the heart rate to normal levels, reduce stress, and help begin the process of recovery.[13] Responsible exercise professionals use both with their clients, and they are generally recommended for everyone. Though they can add a bit of extra time to your daily routine, warm-ups and cool-downs can ultimately eliminate friction by helping you avoid injury. Sustaining an injury that requires taking time off can completely derail a well-established exercise habit.

For most healthy adults, an effective warm-up usually lasts five to ten minutes and includes putting your body through the same motions that you're about to engage in during your primary workout but with light intensity.[14] For example, if your workout for the day includes barbell squats and dumbbell rows, you could warm up with one to two sets of body-weight squats and light resistance band rows. A good warm-up should get the blood flowing to your muscles and make you feel comfortable and ready to perform at a higher intensity level. Once you've gotten your heart beating a bit harder and your applicable muscle groups feel warm and loose, you've probably done enough to start your workout. Refer to the warm-up exercises that you selected in chapter 9 to finalize your specific warm-up plans.

A postworkout cool-down should begin right after the completion of your workout and should also last five to ten minutes.[15] Cool-downs normally include a few minutes of very light cardio such as walking and some static (holding for thirty seconds or more) stretches. For example, someone who's daily workout includes shoulder presses and dead lifts might cool down with a few minutes of walking followed by some shoulder, lower back, and hip and hamstring stretches. The idea with static stretching is to relieve tension in the muscle groups just worked. This book doesn't explore the myriad of available stretching options because many resources on this topic are widely available. If you need additional instructions on proper stretching, any book on basic exercise technique can provide them.

Conclusion

At this point you've learned about each of the essential components of designing an effective daily exercise program. You now know how to

- Arrange strength-training exercises into efficient daily workouts
- Integrate cardio into your daily workouts
- Do your workouts in the right order
- Determine the right number of reps and sets to do for each strength exercise
- Pick the right amount of weight or resistance for strength training
- Effectively recover between sets

With all this knowledge, you are ready to develop your individual workout plan and put it into action. These are the initial steps you should follow to get started:

1. Select a workout space in your home.
2. Decide which exercises will be part of your program.
3. Choose the equipment you will purchase.
4. Design your three daily workouts.
5. Purchase your exercise equipment and set up your home gym.
6. Have a notebook or app available to serve as a performance log.
7. Spend one exercise session determining how much resistance to initially use for each exercise.
8. Begin following your new program.

Remember that if you're unable to complete twenty-minute workouts initially, doing fifteen, ten, or even five minutes is better than nothing. Any amount of daily time spent exercising will be helpful in building a habit, you'll be able to build up to twenty-minute sessions. If you're not ready to commit to purchasing equipment, stick with the alternative exercise recommendations that require minimal equipment. You can build up to purchasing more equipment later. Most importantly, don't entertain the idea that the approach being presented won't work for you—it will. There's no more efficient and sustainable method for making effective exercise part of your everyday life. If you want to get the most out of your time and live the best life possible, then start building your daily exercise habit now.

PART 4

The Nuts and Bolts of Diet and Nutrition

Part 4 is all about learning and applying key principles, strategies, and tactics that can help remove friction from dieting and nutrition. It covers the following topics:

- How to build a general nutritional strategy based on your fitness goals
- Strategies for selecting calorie- and nutrient-efficient foods
- How to build a core meal plan
- Efficient methods for tracking and managing your diet

By the end of this section, you'll know how to leverage the key ideas for removing friction from the meal-building process, minimize tedious calorie counting, recover when you slip up or have a cheat day, and most importantly, how to make effective nutritional planning and dieting a lifelong habit.

Note that the scope and purpose of this section is to teach some key principles that can help remove friction from the dieting and meal-planning process. Though it does provide examples of meal plans and references certain types of food, it does so only to provide examples of friction-reducing principles being applied to realistic but hypothetical scenarios. This section is in no way endorsing a particular type of diet, nor does it recommend eating specific types or quantities of foods or nutrients. All references made in these chapters relating to dietary, food, caloric, and nutrient intake recommendations are based on adult populations in good health. This advice is general, evidence-based, and meant for educational purposes only. If you are looking for a personalized meal plan or grocery list, you should consult the services of a registered dietitian or other qualified nutrition professional. Any choices that you make about the contents of your specific diet or meal plan should be based on the latest scientific evidence from accredited academic, scientific, or government sources.

CHAPTER 12

Diet and Nutrition Basics

AFTER BUILDING YOUR EXERCISE PROGRAM, you can now start to grasp the important role that nutrition and diet play in your overall health and fitness. The term *nutrition* refers to the organic compounds that food is made of. The term *diet* refers to the foods that you rely on for nutrition, specifically, the types and quantities of those foods. In other words, nutrition is what the body needs, and diet is how the body gets it. Having a fundamental understanding of both fields and building positive habits from that knowledge is essential to maintaining and improving long-term physical fitness. This chapter lays the initial groundwork you'll need for designing, implementing, and sustaining an effective and efficient nutritional and dietary plan.

The Relationship between Nutrition, Diet, and Exercise

Before all else, you need to recognize the relationship between nutrition, diet, and exercise. Though they are different components of fitness, they must function as an integrated system to develop and support a healthy body. Neglecting any one of them has direct negative consequences and can also cause damaging indirect effects. First, let's look at how each component directly supports your overall health.

Nutrition

Eating the right types and amounts of nutrients provides you with the necessary material and resources for maintaining appropriate body composition and chemistry. It ensures the proper functioning of the brain, vital organs, and immune system, and it supports your ability to recover from physical exertion.

Diet

Identifying foods with the right types and amounts of nutritional content enables the body to avoid unhealthy nutrient deficiencies or surpluses. This allows for the development and maintenance of a physically fit body.

Exercise

Proper exercise exhausts your muscles of fuel and can cause structural muscular damage. The body uses the nutrients provided by your diet to refuel and repair any damage—which leads to stronger muscles and more efficient functioning.

Here are some of the ways that neglecting any one of these critical fitness disciplines can negatively impact all three areas.

Inadequate Nutrition

Failing to eat foods with the right nutritional content makes it difficult to fuel bodily processes or repair muscular damage incurred during physical activity. This means that performance during workouts will be harder and improving fitness will be more difficult.

Poor Diet

Undereating results in inadequate nutrition, which can ultimately be life threatening. The overeating of foods—even healthy ones—leads to increased body fat and an increased risk of disease. Being overweight—a direct effect of poor diet—makes exercise more difficult, primarily by limiting mobility.

Inadequate Exercise

Lack of exercise directly undercuts your ability to cultivate and maintain a fit body. Fitness can be achieved and sustained only by regularly putting adequate stress on the muscles so they can recover and strengthen. Appropriate nutrition and diet provide the energy and material necessary for this process to work. But without adequate exercise, the potential positive effects of both become much more limited. Inadequate or total lack of exercise reduces the benefits that eating right can provide.

Each discipline can deliver its full benefits only when proper nutrition, diet, and exercise are practiced together as a unified system. For this reason, have a sustainable and healthy diet and nutritional plan to support your exercise system.

Key Components of Nutrition

The first step to developing healthy eating patterns is grounding yourself in the basics of nutrition. You don't have to be an expert, but you need a rudimentary understanding of what's important and what's not. As with exercise science, the science of nutrition is an ever-expanding field that's rapidly making new discoveries, so be willing to incorporate new recommendations into your system if they add value. Though the available information on nutrition is constantly increasing, *some* fundamental components aren't likely to change. The exploration of nutrition presented in this chapter is limited to these fundamentals. Sticking to the basics allows for system flexibility and avoids the trap of making final judgments on controversial topics that science hasn't yet settled. If you build a plan on the fundamentals, you'll be positioned to expand and enhance your system as your knowledge of diet and nutrition increases over time.

As was said in chapter 6, all the food you eat is made up of substances called macronutrients (a.k.a. macros). They are divided into three subcategories: proteins, carbohydrates, and fats. These three macros plus hydration are the four basic building blocks of human nutrition. Most of the complexity and debate over nutrition relates to macros—specifically, what foods are the best sources of macros and how much of each to eat. What's generally not debated is that the human body needs adequate amounts of all these building blocks to function properly. By learning the basic attributes of each, you'll begin understanding how they work together to sustain your body. Below are some brief descriptions of each type of macro and some examples of various foods that contain them.

Protein

Protein is a primary building block of your body that is used to build and repair tissues and make hormones and other chemicals, and it is an essential component of your blood, skin, hair, nails, bones, organs, muscle, and cartilage. Excluding water and fat, the human body is made almost entirely of protein. Proteins themselves are composed of smaller components called *amino acids*, which link together into long chains. Some amino acids—known as *essential amino acids*—can't be produced by the body, so we must get them from food. Protein is primarily used to build and repair body tissue, break down food, and perform many other important functions. An especially unique characteristic of protein is that—unlike fat and carbohydrates—it can't be stored by the body for future use. Excess protein generally gets converted into fat and cannot be transformed back to protein later.[1] This means that your body needs to take in new protein frequently and consistently for proper functioning.

The two basic sources of dietary protein come from animals and plants. Some common examples of animal proteins are lean meat, poultry, fish, eggs, milk, yogurt, and cheese. Some common examples of plant-based proteins are nuts, seeds, beans, legumes, and soy products.[2]

For general health in most adults, the current recommended daily allowance (RDA) for protein is 10 to 35 percent of the total daily calorie intake.[3] If, for example, people eating 2,000 calories per day were following a diet that is 10 percent protein, they'd need to eat 200 protein calories per day (which is 50 grams of protein). Note that people who are physically active or reducing their calorie intake to lose weight will require more protein.[4] The recommended protein intake ranges for most people trying to maximize muscle development are as follows:

- For men: 0.9–1.18 grams of protein per pound of lean body mass
- For women: 0.82–1.0 gram of protein per pound of lean body mass

Eating substantially more protein beyond these ranges doesn't seem to aid further muscle development.[5] Also, notice that the recommended protein ranges for maximal muscle development are based on lean body mass (LBM), which you learned to calculate in chapter 5. To calculate daily protein intake based on these recommended ranges, multiply your LBM by an amount of protein (in grams) in the specified range for your sex. For example, Sarah weighs 140 pounds and has an LBM of 112 pounds. She plans to eat one gram of protein per pound of lean mass, so she'd eat 112 grams of protein per day (at her current weight) to help maximize muscle development.

Carbs

For most people, carbohydrates (a.k.a. carbs) serve as the body's main source of energy, and they come in three primary varieties: fiber, starch, and sugar. Through digestion, carbs are converted into glucose—blood sugar—which is then used by cells, tissues, and organs for energy. Glucose is primarily absorbed by the liver and muscles for fuel, but if not used, it's ultimately stored as fat.[6]

Be aware of the variation that can occur in the structure of carbs. Carbs have two basic types of structure: simple and complex. Simple carbs are sugar based and are primarily found in processed foods such as sodas, candies, baked sweets, breakfast cereals, and juice from concentrate, but they also occur naturally in some foods. These carbs are broken down quickly, delivering a quick burst of energy, but this energy is rapidly depleted—an occurrence known as a *sugar crash*. The simple carbs found in processed foods—such as refined sugar—also lack important vitamins and minerals. This is why they're often referred to as having "empty calories"—because they have limited nutritional value. The notable exceptions are foods with naturally occurring simple carbs such as milk and fruits—they generally *do* contain essential vitamins and nutrients.[7]

Complex carbs come in two varieties: starches and dietary fiber. They perform two very different functions, both of which are important in a healthy diet. Starches are made up of long chains of sugar molecules, which take more time to digest. They don't cause the sudden bursts of energy—and subsequent sugar crashes—that can come with eating simple carbs. Common foods such as whole wheat bread, corn, rice, and oats are high in starches. Dietary fibers are plant based and predominantly indigestible carbs, which pass through the digestive system relatively unchanged. They help with bowel health, lower cholesterol, control blood sugar levels, and keep you feeling full. Some common foods high in fiber are fruits, vegetables, nuts, beans, and whole grains.[8]

For general health in most adults, the current RDA for carbs is 45 to 65 percent of the total daily calorie intake.[9] If, for example, people eating 2,000 calories per day were following a diet that is 60 percent carbs, they'd need to eat 1,200 carb calories per day (which is 300 grams of carbs). Note that while the body doesn't require carbs to create glucose, eating a moderate amount of carbs is generally advised for enhanced exercise performance, especially when a person's goal is to maximize muscle development. Current research hasn't conclusively defined an ideal carb intake for maximizing muscle development, but a minimum intake of about 1.36 grams per pound of total body mass seems to be a reasonable amount. For example, Brian weighs 185 pounds and plans to eat 1.36 grams of carbohydrates for every pound of his body weight, so he'd be eating about 252 grams of carbs daily (which is 1,008 calories). Note that individual carb requirements may vary due to a variety of factors, so personal preference and bodily response to training may warrant higher intake levels.[10]

Also note that your muscle development goal can have a significant influence on the amount of carbs that you choose to eat. If your goal is to gain weight by maximizing muscle development, then 1.36 grams of carbs per pound of body weight is a reasonable starting place. If, however, your goal is to maintain muscle mass and body weight, or maintain muscle while losing body fat, then your carb intake may need to be lower to maintain an energy balance or calorie deficit. In the latter situations, you can defer to the current carbohydrate RDA of 45 to 65 percent of your daily caloric intake.

Fats

Dietary fat is often spoken of in a negative context, but it's absolutely required by our bodies for proper functioning. Fat is primarily used as an energy source and to help absorb fat-soluble vitamins (A, D, E, and K). Excess fat is stored in fat cells, which provides energy reserves as well as warmth and insulation. The fat in foods provides us with essential fatty acids that the body can't create on its own. These essential acids are needed for brain health, the regulation of inflammation, and blood clotting.[11]

The three primary types of dietary fat are saturated, trans, and unsaturated. Saturated fats usually come from animal sources such as red meat, poultry, and full-fat dairy and are solid at room temperature (e.g., butter). Certain plant products such as palm and coconut oil are also saturated fats. Too much saturated fat is generally considered to be unhealthy because it raises LDL (bad) cholesterol levels, which can build up in arteries. Trans fats are mostly found in processed foods, though they do naturally occur in some whole foods (such as red meat) in small amounts. The processed types are made by turning liquid oils into solid products such as margarine or shortening. Trans fats raise LDL (bad) cholesterol levels and lower HDL (good) cholesterol, which increases the risk of heart disease and stroke. Your body does not need trans fats, so most foods containing them should be avoided.[12]

Unsaturated fats (a.k.a. good fats) are liquid at room temperature and mainly come from plants, nuts, seeds, and fish. They are known to raise HDL (good) cholesterol, lower LDL cholesterol, and fall into one of two main categories—monounsaturated or polyunsaturated. Polyunsaturated fats contain the essential fatty acids required by the body for critical functioning and can be found in common foods such as flaxseed, walnuts, and fatty fish; they're also found in sunflower, corn, soybean, and canola oils. They have also been linked to the prevention of heart disease and strokes, and they generally promote cardiovascular health. Monosaturated fats are also associated with lower rates of heart disease and can be found in common foods such as avocados; nuts; and olive, canola, sunflower, and peanut oils.[13]

For general health in most adults, the current RDA for fat is 20 to 35 percent of the total daily calorie intake.[14] If, for example, people eating 2,000 calories per day were following a diet that is 20 percent fat, they'd need to eat 400 fat calories per day (which is about 44 grams of fat). Current research has yet to define ideal fat intake guidelines for maximizing muscle development, but generally, the balance of your daily calories can be allocated to fat after accounting for protein and carbs. A minimum of 0.45 grams of fat per pound of total body mass seems to be enough to prevent hormonal changes that can negatively impact muscle development. For example, Bethany weighs 155 pounds and plans to eat 0.45 grams of fat for every pound of her body weight, so she'd be eating about 70 grams of fat daily (which is 630 calories). To further enhance muscle development, evidence suggests prioritizing unsaturated fats—particularly polyunsaturated fats—over saturated fats.[15]

Hydration

The importance of water cannot be understated; water is so crucial to vital functioning that just a few days without any will cause death. It generally accounts for two-thirds of a person's total mass and is required by every organ and cell for proper functioning. Here's just a sampling of the important tasks that water does in our bodies: regulates temperature, lubricates joints, flushes waste out of the kidneys and liver, dissolves minerals and organic compounds for absorption, and carries nutrients and oxygen to cells for use. Dehydration is detrimental to virtually all bodily processes, including exercise. Without proper hydration, you won't be able to function properly during workouts or recover properly afterward.[16] You must consistently drink enough water to develop and maintain a healthy body.

The amount of fluid you should drink varies by individual, but the general recommendations from the National Academies of Sciences, Engineering, and Medicine is eleven and a half cups per day for women and fifteen and a half cups per day for men.[17] This advice is generally good, but your body weight and activity level effect the amount of fluid you need.

The most effective hydration strategy is to aim for these targets by drinking water over the course of the day while watching for signs of dehydration. Water is excreted every time you sweat or urinate, which can cause gradual dehydration if you're not regularly replenishing fluids. The best way to detect dehydration is by looking at the color of your urine. If you're urinating every two to four hours and the urine is light colored, then you're hydrated.[18] If you're urinating less often and the urine is a darker yellow color, you're dehydrated. In the latter situation, you'd need to increase your fluid intake, even if you'd already met the fluid intake recommendation. After a few days of observation, you'll gain a much better idea of what's necessary to keep your body hydrated.

Water generally isn't the sole source of fluid in a person's diet; other foods and beverages also contribute to hydration. Drinks such as milk, juices, and sodas are just as effective as water, but be mindful of the caloric and nutritional content of these alternatives. Many of these beverages are especially high in sugar. Contrary to popular belief, caffeinated drinks such as coffee and tea also help with rehydration despite their tendency to cause more frequent urination. Even some fruits and vegetables can help replenish fluids due to their higher water content. Some notable examples are melons, oranges, grapefruit, celery, cucumbers, tomatoes, and lettuce.[19] While drinking water should be your primary means of hydrating, be sure to take all relevant fluid sources into account as you build a hydration plan.

Vitamins (Micronutrients)

The final type of nutrients that must be discussed are called micronutrients, or vitamins and minerals. These nutrients are deemed essential for good health because they play an important role in many vital processes such as immune health, brain function, overall body growth, bone health, and fluid balance. Our bodies can't produce most micronutrients, so we must get them from dietary sources.[20] Ideally, you'll get adequate micronutrients from eating a variety of unprocessed foods, but being deficient of some micronutrients is relatively common. If you're deficient, improving your fitness can be more difficult. The two possible solutions are changing your diet or taking dietary supplements. The only way to determine whether you have a deficiency is by having blood work done. Annual physicals with your physician are a good time to discuss micronutrients because you'll generally be having your blood analyzed at that time. Asking your doctor if your micronutrient levels are normal during these checkups is a good idea. If you have any deficiencies, he or she will be able to recommend an appropriate dietary change or regimen of vitamin supplements.

Building a Nutritional Plan

Now that you have a good foundational understanding of what the body requires for sustenance, you are ready to build a nutritional plan tailored to your goals. To do this, make four important determinations:

- How many calories you'll eat per day
- How many grams of protein you'll eat per day
- How many grams of fat you'll eat per day
- How many grams of carbs you'll eat per day

Your daily calorie target represents the total amount of food that you'll eat in a twenty-four-hour period. Your protein, fat, and carb targets represent how much of each type of macro you'll eat during that time. Note that the calorie content of the protein, fat, and carbs you consume *all* contribute to your total daily calorie count. Table 12.1 shows how many calories each type of macronutrient contains.

The most important part of building a proper nutritional plan is determining the right combination of macros to eat. Doing so ensures that your diet provides adequate nutrients *and* the right number of calories. The two ways to accomplish this are

- You can use a macronutrient calculator tool to make the calculations for you.
- You can calculate your plan manually based on your body-composition metrics.

Using a calculator tool is quick (usually taking less than five minutes), and it provides a solid general plan. Making the calculations manually takes more time (up to one hour) but can be helpful when more customization is desired. Most people use a calculator to build an initial plan. You can revisit your nutrition plan later and learn to manually calculate new targets if you want.

Table 12.1
Caloric Content of Macronutrients

MACRONUTRIENT	GRAMS	CALORIES
Protein	1	4
Fat	1	9
Carbs	1	4

Using a Macro Calculator Tool

A good macro calculator uses your age, sex, height, weight, activity level, weight goal, and macronutrient intake preferences to automatically generate a nutritional plan based on population averages and evidence-based data. You simply plug in your information, and the tool will give a daily calorie goal and a target for each macro. The easiest solution is to use the calculator available on my website. Go to frictionfactorfitness.com to access it.

When you use a nutrition calculator, be sure to set the correct activity level and weight goal. Since you'll be following the twenty-minute-per-day exercise strategy, your activity level will probably be in the one-to-three-hours-per-week range—unless you have a physically demanding job. When entering a body-weight goal into the tool, remember that people trying to reduce body fat should aim for no more than two pounds of weight loss per week. Likewise, those trying to gain mass should aim for no more than one to two pounds of weight gain per week.[21]

Once you've entered all your information, the tool will generate a nutritional profile for you. Tables 12.2 and 12.3 offer examples of nutritional plans generated by the calculator tool.

Good nutrition plans don't stay completely static over time. This means that you can't use a macro calculator once and then follow that same plan forever. As your body composition changes, so do your nutrient requirements. For instance, if you determine that you need 1,700 calories per day to lose weight at a rate of one pound per week, this will hold true at only your current body weight. Once you've lost a few pounds, your calorie requirements will be different. To continue losing weight at the same rate (one pound per week), you will need to recalculate your plan at your lower body weight.

If you're trying to gain weight, your nutrient requirements will likewise change as you build mass. At your current weight, you might

Table 12.2

Sample Nutritional Profile 2: Male

Age	35
Weight	200
Height (inches)	70
Body mass goal	Weight loss 1.5 lb per week
Activity level	Light activity (1 to 3 hours of exercise per week)
Protein target (grams/day)	150
Fat target (grams/day)	41
Carb target (grams/day)	195
Total daily calories	1,745

Table 12.3

Sample Nutritional Profile 1: Female

Age	38
Weight	145
Height (inches)	65
Body mass goal	Weight loss 1 lb per week
Activity level	Light activity (1 to 3 hours of exercise per week)
Protein target (grams/day)	96
Fat target (grams/day)	38
Carb target (grams/day)	146
Total daily calories	1,307

need to eat two hundred to three hundred more calories per day to put on size. Once you put on a few pounds, you will need to recalculate your calorie target because your requirements for further gains will change as you become heavier. If you're trying to gain or lose weight, come back and recalculate your plan every two weeks or so, especially if your body weight has changed by a few pounds. The only scenario when regular recalculation isn't necessary is when you're trying to maintain your current mass and body composition.

If you haven't already done so, use the macro calculator to calculate your initial nutritional plan. Once your plan is defined, you're ready to begin meal planning—which is covered in the next chapter.

Conclusion

In this chapter, you learned about the fundamental relationship between nutrition, diet, and exercise and why all three components must function as an integrated system to develop and support a fit body. You now have a basic understanding of the roles of protein, carbohydrates, and fats in human nutrition and what the current recommended intake levels are for each. You've learned about the importance of hydration and how to ensure that you're staying hydrated. You've also learned about micronutrients and why regularly having blood work done is important so your doctor can help address any deficiencies or overages. Finally, you learned the basic steps of building a nutritional plan and how to use a macro calculator to simplify the process of creating an initial nutrient intake plan. By learning about the important role that nutrition and diet play in physical fitness, you've begun laying the groundwork for designing, implementing, and sustaining an effective and efficient nutritional and dietary strategy.

CHAPTER 13

Preparing for Meal Planning

THIS CHAPTER WILL BUILD ON the information on nutrition you've learned to help you prepare for effective and efficient meal planning by covering the following topics:

- Core daily meals and staple foods
- How to select calorie-efficient staple foods
- How many meals to eat per day
- How to calculate per-meal macronutrient targets

Core Daily Meals and Staple Foods

Once you've determined a daily calorie budget and set macronutrient targets, you'll need to determine what foods to eat. This can be difficult because you probably don't have the time every day to translate calorie and macronutrient goals into real meals and grocery lists. For most people, the idea of reading food labels, counting every calorie, and doing math on your napkin after each meal is a major deterrent to eating right. This is totally understandable because traditional calorie counting and meal planning take significant time and energy. One of the main reasons people can't make healthy dieting a habit is that they don't have the available bandwidth to fit it into their busy life. This is also why people revert to their old unhealthy eating patterns when life gets hectic—because following bad habits is easier than making new habits. When your time and energy are limited, dietary plans that require significant thinking and decision-making simply create too much friction.

How can a busy person begin implementing an effective diet plan? The first step is realizing that when you don't have much free time to devote to dieting, the primary enemy of success is complexity. Beginners often give themselves far too many food options for what to eat; they also tend to select options that take too much time to prepare. Once you know your daily macro targets, construct meals that allow you to easily meet those targets. With too many food options, you end up with an overwhelming number of potential meal plans to manage. This presents people with a difficult puzzle to solve every time they need to eat. When the meals you've selected are also time consuming and tedious to prepare, you add even more steps to the process of satiating hunger. All this complexity quickly becomes a hurdle when you don't have much time or energy to put toward dieting. When you're hungry and short on time—which is often the case—you need a low-friction solution. Your meals need to be nutritious, satisfying, quick to prepare, and easily accessible. Any dieting plan that doesn't meet these requirements is almost certain to fail.

The easiest way to simplify the dieting process is to rely primarily on three to five core daily meals to meet your macronutrient and calorie requirements. By consistently consuming these core meals with fixed portion sizes and nutrient content, you eliminate the need to make lots of decisions every time you eat. This notion should ring familiar because the approach is identical to my approach to exercise (i.e., that your exercise program should be composed of core daily workouts). In the case of dieting, high-friction activities, such as label reading and calorie counting, can be eliminated by mostly relying on a predesigned set of core meals. As with core workouts, designing a core system of repeatable meals takes some upfront work. But once your meal plan is built, it can be automated so that no major thinking or decision-making is required on an everyday basis.

To develop effective core meals, identify a few primary sources of protein, fat, and carbs to serve as your main nutritional building blocks. These building blocks are referred to as *staple foods* in this book. Having staples eliminates friction in the meal-planning process by narrowing the overwhelming range of options for macronutrient sources. Taking this approach also allows you to think about building meals in terms of specific food types versus thinking in terms of calories and macros.

In some distant future, perhaps, we'll all have three tubes sticking out of our kitchen walls that dispense pure protein, fat, and carbs (which would all taste delicious). We could preprogram these tubes to squirt out the appropriate amount of each macronutrient for every meal, making dieting completely effortless. Unfortunately, this vision is currently science fiction. Today we must comb grocery-store shelves and scrutinize nutrition labels to find appropriate food sources. The closest we can come to the simplicity of the three tubes is building meals with staple foods. Your staples will be your food tubes that make meal planning as easy as possible.

Staple Food Considerations

The primary qualifications for an effective staple food are appropriate nutritional content, accessibility, affordability, and satiation. In other words, good staples must meet your macro requirements, be easy to attain and prepare, be affordable, and satisfy your hunger. To guide you through the process of selecting staples, we'll explore some important considerations to make and survey some great staple options. In most cases, choosing a few different staples rich in each type of macro is best. For instance, you might have a primary staple protein food and then one or two alternate proteins in your arsenal. This approach is helpful because factors such as when and where you eat your meals can often make some food options impractical. The fewer staple foods you choose, the less complex it will be to manage your nutrition.

Calorie-Efficient Foods

As you consider potential staple food options, pay special attention to how efficiently a given food can deliver the desired type of macro. Generally, you'll want to consider foods with a relatively high proportion of a *single* type of macro. The broad guidelines for selecting calorie-efficient staple foods are as follows:

- Ideal staple proteins are *high* in protein and *low* in carbs and fat.
- Ideal staple carbs are *high* in carbohydrates and *low* in protein and fat.
- Ideal staple fats are *high* in fat and *low* in protein and carbs.

Here are a few examples of calorie-efficient foods:

- Tuna is a great staple protein option because about 89 percent of its calories come from protein—which is very high.
- Sweet potatoes are an extremely efficient staple carb option because about 94 percent of their calories come from carbs.
- Extra virgin olive oil is an efficient staple fat option because 100 percent of its calories come from fat.

By selecting calorie-efficient staple foods, you'll make it much easier to design meals with the right number of calories and nutrients to hit your targets.

The foods listed in tables 13.1, 13.2, and 13.3 show more common examples of calorie-efficient foods, but this book is not advocating that your meals should be composed of these specific foods. These examples were selected to help further your grasp of the principle of calorie efficiency, and they are by no means the only options. You can find many other staple food options beyond those listed by searching the internet using terms such as

- Healthy foods high in protein
- Healthy foods high in fat
- Healthy foods high in carbs

Your search results should show most of the macro content and calorie information you need. If not, that data can be at your fingertips in seconds with a food-specific search query:

- How much protein is in a chicken breast?
- How many calories are in a chicken breast?

If you want professional and more-personalized assistance selecting appropriate staple foods, consider temporarily hiring a registered dietician (RD). An RD should be able to help you build a great list of staple food options tailored to your specific situation and goals.

Selecting your staple foods should not be a separate activity from building each of your core daily meals—breakfasts, lunches, dinners, and snacks. For instance, don't deem steak your staple protein until you've considered the types of meals you want and what your fat and carb sources might be. Taking this wider perspective is critical because the various types of staples you select can impact the types of meals you'll be able to construct. The following three sections are about selecting proteins, carbs, and fats. Then it will be explained how to apply that information to the meal-building process.

Protein Staples

When it comes to maintaining muscle mass and enhancing muscle development, protein is the macro that the average person struggles to consume enough of. This happens for a few reasons. First, people struggle to get enough protein because it's generally the most expensive of the three macronutrients, so people tend to buy inadequate supplies of it. Second, many good protein sources require a significant amount of time to prepare. For example, if you're hungry for a hamburger, you might have to defrost the meat, then season it, and then cook it—which can take some time. People often turn to carb- or fat-based meals when they're hungry because they can generally be prepared much faster.

If you're like most people, you don't have unlimited funds for food, so you need to be strategic in selecting your protein sources. Since protein is generally the most expensive macronutrient, select your protein staples first. See table 13.1 for a sample list of common foods high in protein and their nutritional content. Once you've allocated funds for protein, you can then determine what carbs and fats to buy.

Table 13.1
Protein Source Examples

Food	Protein (per-cent)	Protein content (grams)	Total calories	Average price rating	Prep time
Canned tuna (8 oz)	89	40	180	$	Low
Shrimp (8 oz)	84	47.4	225	$$$	High
Whey protein powder (32 g)	80	25.3	126	$$	Low

Table 13.1 *(continued)*

Food	Protein (Percent)	Protein Content (Grams)	Total Calories	Average Price Rating	Prep Time
Chicken breast (8 oz)	75	70.4	374	$$	High
Salmon (8 oz)	69	58	338	$$$	High
Low-fat Greek yogurt (8 oz)	67	22.7	136	$	Low
Fat-free cottage cheese (8 oz)	65	26.2	161	$	Low
Hemp protein powder (8 oz)	53	64	480	$$	Low
93 percent lean turkey breast (8 oz)	47	40	340	$$	Medium
Soy tempeh (3 oz)	45	18	160	$$$	Medium
Lean sirloin steak (8 oz)	42	60.8	583	$$$	High
85 percent lean beef (8 oz)	41	58.8	567	$$	Medium
Eggs (2 large)	34	12	140	$	Medium

Selecting your proteins first is also good for helping you stay within your calorie plan. First, you need to determine how many of your allotted daily calories will be consumed in the form of protein. Then, the remaining number of unassigned calories will help narrow the scope for what foods are viable carb and fat options. For instance, Corey's daily calorie limit is 2,000, his macro target for protein is 120 grams, and his staple protein is ground turkey. He needs to eat about 1,000 calories of turkey each day to get his protein—which leaves 1,000 calories remaining for carbs and fats.

In addition to affordability, also consider how and when you will be consuming your meals. If you have enough free time every day to spend an hour or more cooking, you'll have very different food options than people with a busier lifestyle. Ideally, have at least one staple protein available that doesn't require any preparation; some good examples are protein powder, Greek yogurt, and cottage cheese. Each of these foods can be used to make a high-protein meal instantaneously, which can be a lifesaver when you don't have much time.

While having a quick protein staple is extremely important, you probably won't want it to be your single source. Most people prefer their primary staple protein to be some type of meat, seafood, or poultry. Usually these options require more steps to prepare, which means more friction, but you can take steps to minimize the friction. The most notable solution is batch cooking, which entails cooking and portioning all your staple foods for a week during a single weekly prep session.

While batch cooking usually takes a significant amount of time, the payoff is that it makes foods that normally have long prep times viable meal options. For example, Monica's staple protein is ground beef. She prefers to cook several pounds of it in an hour-long session once per week. She then portions the meat into single-meal containers and freezes them for use throughout the week. Whenever she needs a quick meal, she just pulls the prepared protein from storage and heats it up. A tremendous number of books and online resources are available that include batch cooking, so explore the options and find one that fits your situation. Ultimately these techniques and methods are beneficial because they expand the number of potential staple food options available to you.

Fat Staples

Once you've selected a staple protein for a meal, selecting staple fats next is usually best. This is advisable because fats are the most calorie-dense macronutrient at nine calories per gram, as shown in table 13.2.

Your protein sources (especially dairy) will contribute some amount of fat, so account for this before choosing any staple fats. After accounting for any fat that will come from your staple proteins, you may find that you don't have many available calories left to devote to fats. What follows are two examples of how the types of fats a person can choose will vary depending on their macro targets—notice that the daily calorie targets are the same in both examples:

In the first example, Marcus is on a low-fat 2,000-calorie-per-day diet. His fat target is 45 grams per day, which is 20 percent of his daily calorie intake. His staple proteins per day are two scoops of whey protein powder, 12 ounces of lean ground turkey, and 6 ounces of fat-free cottage cheese. This provides 134 grams of protein spread across his daily meals. In addition to the protein, these staples also contribute 31 grams of fat (and 13 grams of carbs). Marcus only has 14 grams of fat left in his daily budget but still needs to consume nearly 1,000 calories worth of carbs. He needs to add a bit more fat to his diet, so, he adds olive oil to a salad as dressing to get his remaining fat. Marcus needs to get the rest of his calories from foods high in healthy carbs and with little or no fat (such as rice).

In a second example, Jacob is on a high-fat (lower-carb) 2,000-calorie-per-day diet. His fat macro target is 78 grams per day (35

Table 13.2

Fat Source Examples

Food	Fat (percent)	Fat Content (grams)	Total Calories	Average Price Rating	Prep Time
Coconut oil (1 tbsp)	100	13.6	118	$$	Low
Extra virgin olive oil (1 tbsp)	100	13.5	119	$$	Low
Avocado (1)	81	29	322	$$	Low
Peanut butter, plain with no sugar added (2 tbsp)	80	28.3	319	$	Low
Full-fat yogurt (8 oz)	80	13.3	150	$	Low
Almonds (23 nuts)	77	13.6	159	$$	Low
Parmesan cheese (1 oz)	61	2.9	43	$$	Low
Eggs (2)	60	9.5	143	$	Medium
Tofu (4 oz)	48	5.9	111	$$	High
Milk 2 percent (8 oz)	35	4.8	122	$	Low

percent of daily calorie intake). His staple proteins are the same as the previous example: two scoops of whey protein, 12 ounces of ground turkey, and 6 ounces of fat-free cottage cheese—which provide 134 grams of protein. With 31 grams of fat coming from his protein sources, he still needs to get 47 grams of fat (423 fat calories). He also needs to consume over 600 more calories in the form of carbs. Jacob should consider eating higher quantities of foods that are rich in healthy fats such as seeds, nuts, and soybean products. He'd need these types of foods to get the fat that he requires.

As you can see, the types of staple fats that you choose can vary widely depending on your macro goals. Regardless of whether you're following a high-fat, low-fat, or moderate-fat plan, try to prioritize eating more unsaturated fats, limit saturated fats, and stay away from trans fats.

Carb Staples

When selecting your staple carb sources—which should be done after proteins and fats have been selected—your primary concern should be food quality. Most foods on grocery-store shelves are packed with carbohydrates, but few of them are healthy choices. Most of these foods are processed, meaning they're composed of simple carbs and provide no additional vitamins or minerals. In nearly every case, the healthiest carbs come from whole foods—which don't contain additives (such as sugary syrups) and have not been processed. Notice that all the foods listed in table 13.3 are whole fruits, vegetables, or grains. These types of foods contain the complex carbs you should be using to fuel your body. Prioritize staple carb sources that fall into this category.

The composition of many carb-rich foods is varied. An implication of this is that you won't be able to get everything you need from one carb source. Also note that some carb-rich foods—such as pasta—also contain fat, so you'll need to account for and adjust your staple

Table 13.3
Carb Source Examples

Food	Carb (percent)	Carb content (grams)	Fiber (grams)	Total calories	Average price rating	Prep time
Apples (8 oz)	99	29.25	5.5	118	$	Low
Carrots (1 medium)	96	6	1.7	25	$	Low
Sweet potatoes (8 oz)	94	45.6	6.8	195	$	High
Bananas (8 oz)	94	47.5	6	202	$	Low
Oatmeal (8 oz)	88	58.8	3.9	266	$	Low
White rice (8 oz)	88	53.2	0.6	218	$	High
Plain granola (8 oz)	84	79.9	15.6	379	$	Low
Wheat bread (2 slices)	83	25	10	120	$	Low
Green beans (8 oz)	81	7.5	1	37	$	Low

Table 13.3 *(continued)*

Food	Carb (per-cent)	Carb con-tent (grams)	Fiber (grams)	Total calo-ries	Aver-age price rating	Prep time
Kidney beans (8 oz)	80	44	16.8	220	$	Medium
Red bell pepper (1 cup chopped)	78	9	3.1	46	$	Low
Peas (8 oz)	72	21	11	117	$	Medium
Quinoa (8 oz)	71	48.3	5.2	272	$$	High
Spinach (8 oz)	49	6.37	4.3	52	$$	Low

fat quantities if you select carbs with a significant fat content. Here are some helpful facts about the primary types of carbohydrates:

- Dark green vegetables are high in vitamin K.
- Red and orange vegetables are high in vitamin A.
- Beans, peas, and lentils are high in fiber.
- Starchy vegetables are high in potassium.
- Fruits are high in fiber, potassium, and vitamin C.
- Whole grains contain several important nutrients including iron, zinc, magnesium, and vitamin B6.

The current general recommendation for a healthy dietary pattern is to include a variety of foods in your plan across these different categories.[2] Here are a few more helpful thoughts, strategies, and tactics for selecting staple carbs:

Fruits—Fruits give a quick energy source. They're great for before and after workouts as well as for a pick-me-up snack. They're also highly transportable and require no preparation.

Green leafy vegetables—Green leafy vegetables are a low-calorie source of fiber and vitamins and are an easy way to add additional nutrition to your meals with little effort. They can be eaten alongside a protein as a salad, quickly steamed (even in a microwave), or added to blended drinks, such as protein shakes or smoothies.

Starches and grains—Unless you rely heavily on fat as a primary energy source, you'll need some other energy source to go along with your protein, and starches are great for this. You can't rely completely on fruit for carbs because too much fruit may have a negative effect on blood sugar levels. You also can't rely too heavily on leafy greens because they're so low in calories, you'd have to eat a ridiculous amount of them to get adequate fuel.

As with protein, prep time is an important factor that should be kept in mind when you're selecting staple carbs. If you usually don't have much time for meal prep, then stay focused on quick options. Most fruits don't require any prep nor do many greens, such as spinach, kale, and lettuce. Some whole grain foods, such as healthy cereals and breads, also don't require preparation. On the other hand, foods such as rice and potatoes cannot be eaten raw and can take a significant amount of time to cook. If you're going to select staple carb options with long prep times, consider batch cooking them so they're readily available throughout the week. As a best practice, even the most diligent batch cooker should have an off-the-shelf carb option in case his or her meal-prep plans fall through.

Number of Daily Meals

After learning the basic considerations to make when selecting staple foods (caloric efficiency, prep time, cost, etc.), the next step is to begin constructing your core daily meals. Again, selecting staple foods while you're designing each meal rather than selecting staples as a separate activity is best. For example, when considering your breakfast meal, you should ask yourself,

- What will be my breakfast protein?
- What will be my breakfast fat?
- What will be my breakfast carbs?

You may use the same staple foods in multiple meals, but selecting staples as you build each meal allows you to make decisions in the right context.

The first question to consider when planning core meals is, How many meals per day will I eat? At one extreme, some people advocate eating five to six small meals throughout the day. At the other extreme, others support intermittent fasting (i.e., eating only one or two large meals during a twenty-four-hour window). No single approach is optimal for everyone, so until science demonstrates otherwise, defer to what's most practical for you. To determine this, look at the flow of your average day and decide where the natural stopping points are. You also need to consider when you typically start feeling hungry and low on energy. If you tend to feel hungry in the morning, then you should eat breakfast. If you're not hungry upon rising, then wait until later to eat. The key principle is to distribute your food intake across however many meals are necessary to keep you feeling full and energized.

Avoid eating meals that don't contain some portion of each of the three macronutrient types. In other words, you shouldn't be eating meals that consist of just protein, just fat, or just carbohydrates. Including some quantity of all three macronutrients in every meal is best because each perform specific functions and provide significant benefits. In general, you should aim to get *all* those benefits from each meal so you spend as much time as possible feeling and operating at your best.

For many people, the old-fashioned three-meal-per-day strategy will be the most practical approach because the flow of virtually everyone's workday has somewhat convenient times for eating in the morning, midday, and evening. Taking meals during these stopping points tends to help with satiation by evenly distributing nutrients across your waking hours. These traditional mealtimes are to some a time-honored custom that gives you some social license to stop what you're doing to eat. Here are a few aspects to consider about each of these customary mealtimes.

Breakfast

In the morning, you've likely gone at least seven to eight hours without eating, which makes breakfast a natural time to refuel. With proper staple food selection and meal planning, anyone can make time for a nutritious breakfast before starting the day. The benefit of eating breakfast is that you're still home in most cases and so have full access to your kitchen and staple foods. You may not have time to cook a formal sit-down meal, but you probably at least have time for something quick, such as Greek yogurt and cereal or a protein shake.

Lunch

The midday meal is a natural stop-and-refuel point because you've likely gone at least four to six hours without food. The other big factor is that most employers still sanction an official lunch break of some kind. People generally take this break, which tends to slow the pace of business and in many cases creates a convenient time to stop and eat.

Dinner

By the evening, you've likely gone another four to six hours without eating and are probably tired from a long day's work. Eating dinner rounds out the day and gives you one last chance to refuel before going to sleep. This is also the most likely point that you'll have some extra time to do more involved meal prep and cooking—which many people enjoy.

Per-Meal Macro Targets

Once you decide what your daily meal frequency will be, you're nearly ready to begin constructing a meal plan. Determine how all your daily calories and macronutrients will be divided across your daily meals. The most important factor is that your total daily consumption of food adds up to meet your calorie and macro targets. While you shouldn't get too hung up on the nutritional contents of any one meal, it is helpful to set per-meal calorie and macro targets. This means aiming to eat a certain number of calories in the form of protein, fat, and carbs during each meal. To set per-meal targets, divide your daily calorie and macro targets by three—or however many meals you're planning to eat daily. Again, don't get too fixated on hitting these targets. Don't worry if, for instance, you prefer a light breakfast but a heavier dinner. The reason for suggesting that you consider evenly distributing nutrients across your meals is that many people find that doing so keeps them feeling more full throughout the day. Tables 13.4 and 13.5 show two different examples of macronutrient distribution plans that include per-meal targets. These examples assume a three-meal-per-day plan but could be easily adjusted for any meal frequency.

Table 13.4

Per-Meal Macro Targets Example 1: Male

Height	5' 10"
Weight (lb)	180
Daily calorie target	2,100
Goal	Weight loss 1 lb per week

Macro targets	Grams	Daily targets Base calories	Percent of total	Per-meal targets (3 meals per day) Grams	Calories
Protein (4 calories/ gram)	144	576	27	48	192
Fat (9 calories/ gram)	56	504	24	19	168
Carb (4 calories/ gram)	255	1,020	49	85	340
Total calories	Total	2,100			700

Table 13.5

Per-Meal Macro Targets Example 2: Female

Height	5' 4"
Weight (lb)	140
Daily calorie target	1,500
Goal	Weight loss 1 lb per week

MACRO TARGETS	DAILY TARGETS			PER-MEAL TARGETS (3 MEALS PER DAY)	
	GRAMS	BASE CALORIES	PERCENT OF TOTAL	GRAMS	CALORIES
Protein (4 calories/ gram)	112	448	30	37	149
Fat (9 calories/ gram)	33	297	20	11	99
Carb (4 calories/ gram)	189	756	50	63	252
Total calories		1,501			500

Conclusion

In this chapter, you learned how to use your newly acquired nutritional knowledge to begin preparing to build an efficient and effective meal plan. You now have a basic understanding of how to select staple foods and use them to construct core meal plans that eliminate friction. You've also learned how to identify calorie-efficient foods and why they should be prioritized as staple foods. Finally, you learned to determine your ideal number of daily meals based on what will keep you full and energized and how to appropriately distribute all your daily nutrients across those meals. After learning about what staple foods are, how to select them, and how they can be used to construct core daily meals, you are now ready to learn the meal-building process.

CHAPTER 14

Building and Managing Your Meal Plan

THIS CHAPTER GOES INTO DETAIL about the critical steps, tips, and tricks for designing, implementing, and sustaining an effective and efficient dieting plan. By the end of it, you'll know how to establish and manage a meal plan while minimizing friction. This chapter covers

- Steps for meal building
- Using nutrition apps to streamline the meal-building process
- How strictly to stick to your diet
- How to efficiently track what you eat
- How to deal with cheat days
- What to eat while traveling

The Meal-Building Process

Once you've calculated your rough per-meal calorie and macro targets, you're almost ready to begin building your core daily meals. As you prepare to start this process, having all your macro targets and calorie goals as well as the example staple food tables from chapter 13 at hand will be helpful when devising meals. In addition, have an internet-capable device available for looking up additional food ideas and nutritional information as needed. Nutrition apps are also invaluable tools for simplifying the meal-building process. The next section will provide specific information regarding when and how to use them. What follows is the step-by-step process you should use to build each of your meals:

1. Select a potential staple food(s) for one of the three macro-nutrients (proteins, fats, or carbs) in the meal, choosing your proteins first.

   For example, if the meal is lunch,
   - Macronutrient: protein
   - Staple food: turkey breast

2. Based on the food's nutritional content, calculate how much of the staple you'd need to eat to hit your macro target for that meal.

   For example, if the staple food is turkey breast, you'll need to note the following nutritional content:
   - Staple food: turkey breast
   - Quantity: 5.6 ounces
   - Protein content: 34 grams
   - Carb content: 0 grams
   - Fat content: 1.4 grams
   - Total calories: 170

3. Is this amount of food reasonable for you to consume or purchase on an ongoing basis? If yes, move on to the next step. If no, go back to step one and select another staple.

- Here's an example: Is this amount of turkey breast reasonable for me to consume/purchase on an ongoing basis?
  - Answer: yes.

4. Does this staple food source align well with your calorie target for this macro? (Keep in mind that even the most calorie-efficient foods will contribute some combination of different macros.) If yes, lock in this staple as a final selection for this meal. If no, consider going back to step one and selecting an alternative staple.

  - For example, ask yourself, Does this staple food source align well with my calorie target for this macro?
  - Answer: yes, my daily target for protein intake is 448 calories.

5. Repeat steps one through four as necessary until you've selected appropriate staple foods and quantities to meet the protein, carb, fat, and calorie requirements of the meal. See table 14.1 for an example.

6. Repeat steps one through five as needed until you've built enough core meal options to satisfy your daily nutrient and calorie targets. See table 14.2 for an example.

Table 14.1

Staple Meal Example

		LUNCH			
FOOD	QUANTITY	PROTEIN (G)	CARBS (G)	FAT (G)	CALORIES
Skinless turkey breast	5.6 oz	34	0	1.4	170
Whole-grain wheat bread	2 slices	10	44	4	240
Tomato	1 slice	0.1	0.6	0	3
Lettuce	2 cups	0.6	2.1	0.1	10
Avocado	2 slices	2	8	14	160
Clementine orange	1 whole	0.6	8.9	0.1	35
Total		47.7	63.5	19.7	618

Table 14.2

Daily Staple Meal-Plan Example

	DAILY TARGETS			PER-MEAL TARGETS (3 MEALS PER DAY)	
MACRO TARGETS	GRAMS	CALORIES	PERCENT OF TOTAL	GRAMS	CALORIES
Protein (4 calories/ gram)	112	448	30	37	149
Fat (9 calories/ gram)	33	297	20	11	99
Carb (4 calories/ gram)	189	756	50	63	252
Total calories		1,500			500

BREAKFAST					
FOOD	QUAN-TITY	PROTEIN (G)	CARBS (G)	FAT (G)	CALORIES
Greek yogurt, plain	6 oz	17	7.9	0	102
Peach, large	1 whole	1.6	16.7	0.4	68
Whole-grain toast	1 piece	5	22	2	120
Butter, unsalted	4 g	0	0	3.2	29
Jam, blackberry	1 tbsp	0	13	0	50
Total		23.6	59.6	5.6	369

continued

Table 14.2 *(continued)*

		LUNCH			
FOOD	QUAN-TITY	PROTEIN (G)	CARBS (G)	FAT (G)	CALORIES
Skinless turkey breast	5.6 oz	34	0	1.4	170
Whole-grain wheat bread	2 slices	10	44	4	240
Tomato	1 slice	0.1	0.6	0	3
Lettuce	2 cups	0.6	2.1	0.1	10
Avocado	2 slices	2	8	14	160
Clementine orange	1 whole	0.6	8.9	0.1	35
Total		47.7	63.5	19.7	618
		DINNER			
FOOD	QUAN-TITY	PROTEIN (G)	CARBS (G)	FAT (G)	CALORIES
Sea scallops	6 oz	28.6	4.5	1.5	151
Roasted mushrooms	0.5 cups	3.5	4.2	4.9	67
Brown rice, cooked	133 g	3.4	30.7	1.2	147
Mixed vegetables	170 g	4	22	0	120
Field greens salad	2 cups	1	2.6	0.1	14
Balsamic vinegar	1 tbsp	0.1	2.7	0	14
Total		40.6	66.7	7.7	513
Daily Total		111.9	189.8	33	1,500

Designing more core meals than you need to get through a given day or week is okay. Some people need variety while others can eat the same foods every day. Just remember that the more options you give yourself, the more complicated the process becomes. Starting with just three to five core daily meals is usually best. You can add more variety over time as you become acclimated to this system.

Sometimes the food choices you make later in planning may require you to adjust some of your earlier selections. For instance, imagine that the staple carb you selected for dinner puts you over your daily calorie limit, but you still want to include it in your meal plan. In this case, you'd need to go back to your plan for breakfast or lunch and make some adjustments so that you don't exceed your calorie target.

Nutrition Apps to Simplify Meal Building

An extremely helpful tool to use throughout the meal-planning process is a digital nutrition app. Many such apps are available for smart phones, tablets, and computers. Most of them even have free versions. I've used one called Lose It! for many years; MyFitnessPal is also a great option. To use a nutrition app to help construct core daily meals, you'll need to utilize the feature that lets users log what they've eaten—nearly all these apps have this option. These meal logs are meant for documenting what you've eaten over the course of a day, but they can also be used for planning hypothetical meals. The idea is to enter a potential breakfast, lunch, and dinner into the log to see whether those meals effectively hit all your daily nutrition targets.

The meal logs in most apps have built-in food libraries that allow you to look up nearly any food imaginable. These libraries allow you to add a food to your meal log and adjust the serving size, and they automatically show the food's nutritional information. The ability to adjust food quantities and automatically see how this affects macros and calories is especially powerful. This function allows you to tinker with your portion sizes to ensure that your meals align with your plan.

For instance, a nutrition app can easily show you how adding an extra four ounces of chicken to your dinner would affect the protein and calorie total for the meal. You would just select baked chicken from the food library and apply four ounces to your meal log. The app would immediately show you how that extra piece of chicken impacts your total daily calories and macros. Trying to calculate your macros and count calories manually simply cannot compete with the speed and flexibility that digital apps provide. Do a little research on available apps and download one—you'll quickly see why they're an indispensable tool for meal planning. The app that you select should be your primary tool for devising core daily meals.

Build Your Meal Plan

You now have the basic information necessary to build a meal plan, so gather all the critical tools and information (a nutrition app and your nutritional plan from chapter 12) and get started! Remember that building your complete meal plan will take some time—maybe even an hour or more, but once the plan is set, it's done. Though you might tweak your plan over time to add variety or because your goals change, the foundation of your meal plan will be solidified. If you stick to your core daily meals, the result will be no more day-to-day guesswork about selecting foods or tedious calorie counting every time you eat.

Seeing sample plans already worked out can be helpful when try-ing to build yours. Take a look at the example core daily meal plans in tables 14.3 and 14.4. They are hypothetical but based on realistic goal profiles.

Table 14.3

Core Daily Meal Plan Example 2: Male

Height	5' 10"
Weight (lb)	180
Daily calorie target	1,643
Goal	Lose 1.5 lb weekly

	DAILY TARGETS			PER-MEAL TARGETS	
MACRO TARGETS	GRAMS	BASE CALORIES	PERCENT OF TOTAL	GRAMS	CALORIES
Protein (4 calories)	137	548	33	46	183
Fat (9 calories)	38	342	21	13	114
Carb (4 calories)	188	752	46	63	251
Total calories		1,642			548

BREAKFAST					
FOOD	QUANTITY	PROTEIN (G)	CARBS (G)	FAT (G)	CALORIES
Shredded wheat cereal	62 g	7.2	49.6	1.6	207
Blueberries	79 g	0.6	11.2	0.3	45
Plain low-fat soy milk	6 oz	3	4.5	1.5	45
100 percent whey protein (shake)	50 g	38.5	2.6	2.6	192
Total		49.3	67.9	6	489

continued

Table 14.3 *(continued)*

		LUNCH			
FOOD	QUANTITY	PROTEIN (G)	CARBS (G)	FAT (G)	CALORIES
Protein bar	1 whole	22	23	7	220
Plant burger patty	1 whole	11	7	0.5	70
Whole wheat hamburger bun	1 whole	3.7	22	2	114
Fat-free hummus	1 tbsp	1	2.5	0	15
Tomato	1 slice	0.1	0.6	0	3
Lettuce	2 slices	1	2	0.2	10
Ketchup	1 tbsp	0.3	3.8	0	15
Total		39.1	60.9	9.7	447

Table 14.3 *(continued)*

		DINNER			
FOOD	QUANTITY	PROTEIN (G)	CARBS (G)	FAT (G)	CALORIES
Iceberg lettuce	2 cups	1	2	0	10
Low-sodium salsa	1 serving	1	4	0	18
Avocado	2 slices	2	8	14	160
Skinless chicken breast	6 oz	33	4.5	4.5	180
Spinach tortilla wrap	1	5	4	1.5	66
Sour cream, low-fat	1.5 tbsp	0.8	1.5	1.9	30
Frozen vegetable medley, cooked	180 g	2.1	10.6	0	64
Brown rice, cooked	161 g	4.1	37.2	1.5	178
Total		49	71.8	23.4	706
Daily total		137.4	200.6	39.1	1,642

Table 14.4

Core Daily Meal Plan Example 2: Female

Height	5' 4"
Weight (lb)	140
Daily Calorie Target	1,545
Goal	Lose 0.5 lb weekly

MACRO TARGETS	DAILY TARGETS			PER-MEAL TARGETS (3 MEALS PER DAY)	
	GRAMS	CALORIES	PERCENT OF TOTAL	GRAMS	CALORIES
Protein (4 calories)	91	364	24	30	121
Fat (9 calories)	34	306	20	11	102
Carb (4 calories)	218	872	56	73	291
Total calories		1,542			514

Table 14.4 (*continued*)

BREAKFAST					
Food	Quantity	Protein (g)	Carbs (g)	Fat (g)	Calories
Black coffee	8 oz	0.3	0	0	2
Medium banana	1	1.3	27	0.4	105
Whole-grain toast	1 piece	5	22	2	120
High-protein cereal	36 g	15.4	10.3	7.7	141
Strawberry fruit spread	1 tbsp	0	3.7	0	30
Total		22	63	10.1	398

LUNCH					
Food	Quantity	Protein (g)	Carbs (g)	Fat (g)	Calories
Whey isolate protein (shake)	29 g	22.9	1.5	7.6	107
Caesar salad	1	3	8	9	120
Sweet potato with skin	7 oz	4	40.8	0.3	180
Light sour cream	1.5 tbsp	0.8	2.3	1.9	30
Apple	1 small	0.4	21	0.3	78
Total		31.1	73.6	19.1	515

continued

Table 14.4 *(continued)*

		DINNER			
FOOD	QUANTITY	PROTEIN (G)	CARBS (G)	FAT (G)	CALORIES
Salmon, grilled	3 oz	27	0	2	150
Garlic and honey sauce	1 tbsp	0	10	0	40
Brown rice, cooked	291 g	7.5	67.2	2.7	322
Mixed vegetables	170 g	4	22	0	120
Total		38.5	99.2	4.6	632
Daily total		91.6	235.8	33.9	1,545

Meal Plan Deviation

Once you've established a set of core daily meals that work for you, you can begin implementing them as your primary source of nutrition. To succeed with the core-meal approach, develop the skill of quickly recovering from instances where you deviate from your plan. Whether you deviate by choice or are forced by circumstances, situations do arise that can make adhering to a meal plan difficult. The question is, How can you make your diet strategy flexible enough to handle occasional deviation and still make progress toward your fitness goals?

First recognize that a one-off "cheat meal" usually won't have much effect on your body composition—even if the meal is heavy. One pound of body fat contains roughly 3,500 calories. While people process calories differently, most people won't eat enough in one meal to put on this much additional body fat. Even if you ate a large 1,200-calorie restaurant dinner—the rough average for Americans—*and* ate cake and ice cream for dessert (another 750 calories), you'd have eaten 1,850 calories total. If your body needed 750 of those calories for energy and protein, then you'd only have eaten an *additional* 1,200 calories. For example, let's assume that your metabolism and core meal plan allow you to lose two pounds per week. The additional 1,200 calories from the cheat meal would probably only have a small negative impact on your weight-loss progress. If you only had one cheat meal that week, you might lose one-and-two-thirds of a pound during the week instead of two—which isn't very significant.

The essential factor for managing the impact of deviations from core meal plans is controlling the frequency of deviation. In other words, people get into trouble with straying from their diet when they do it too often for them to make progress. The challenge is pinpointing the proper threshold, that is, identifying how much deviation from your meal plan is too much. Most people know that they're creating a headwind for themselves when they overeat or have a cheat meal. For an individual meal or a single day, you can even calculate how big of a headwind you've created by counting calories. But calculating the total impact of multiple deviations over longer spans of time and determining their total impact on your fitness progress is difficult. Most people simply don't have time to track everything they eat through manual calorie counting, which is the only method that most people know. Because they don't track exactly what they're eating, determining the feasibility of achieving their fitness goals becomes very difficult.

Let's look at an example of how multiple meal-plan deviations over the course of a week can impact your ability to achieve fitness goals. Brandy is following a core meal plan that should result in one pound of fat loss per week, but she doesn't keep track of her deviations from the plan. Over a seven-day period, she exceeds her daily calorie targets in the following instances:

Monday—Lunch out with her boss: +500 calories
Tuesday—Iced coffee with skim milk: +350 calories
Wednesday—Ice cream cone with the kids: +400 calories
Thursday—Bagel at work: +427 calories
Friday—Popcorn and soda at the movies: +750 calories
Sunday—Family barbecue and birthday cake: +1,100 calories
Total additional calories over seven days: 3,527

Over a whole week, these extra calories result in one pound of fat gain, which completely offsets the one pound Brandy's core meal plan allows her to lose. The result is that she makes no progress toward her fitness goal of reducing body fat. This example demonstrates how just deviating from your meal plan a handful of times each week can make progress toward your fitness goals impossible. This is a problem because when you fail to make progress, your motivation to stick to your fitness plan will start to wear thin.

The Need for Meal Tracking

To allow flexibility into your diet and still have confidence in your ability to make fitness progress, efficiently monitor what you're consuming. Be completely aware of how the food you eat might limit the fitness goals that are attainable for you. The only way to achieve this is by systematically logging and keeping track of everything you consume. Though it may be an uncomfortable truth to hear, every bite of food and sip of a beverage counts and has an impact on body composition. Core meals, an unplanned lunch with friends, or sugar and cream in your coffee all contribute to your calorie intake. Yes, even alcohol counts. A glass of wine, a bottle of beer, or a shot of spirits all have caloric content that should be tracked.

If you don't account for what you eat, you won't see the impact your diet has on your body composition. I'm not suggesting that you never have a cheat meal or drinks with friends. What I do recommend is that you maintain full awareness of the nutritional content of your total diet over time. When you're fully aware of the impact of your food choices, you'll have greater context for deciding when deviating from your meal plan is worth it.

The main difficulty with counting calories and tracking what you eat is that it can be a time-consuming extra step that adds friction to the dieting process. Most people just want to eat their meals and get on with their day without extra hassle. They don't want to manually write down and calculate the calories and macros for everything they eat. The good news is that tracking what you eat is significantly easier today than it was in the past. We've already discussed how to use nutrition apps to build your core meal plan, and using them to keep track of your nutritional intake is also advised. Of course, you can keep a written food diary and manually log meals, but it's not as efficient.

The beauty of using an app to track food consumption is that it drastically reduces the amount of time required to log what you eat. Most apps let you save and copy past meals, which allows you to easily log your core daily meals in a matter of seconds. This means no entering of individual foods or quantities; once a core meal has been entered, it just takes a few clicks to add it to any day's meal log. This is a huge timesaver because your core meals are usually what you'll be eating. The only time that logging your foods can be a bit more involved is when you deviate from your meal plan. Even still, nutrition apps make this much easier. The robust food libraries in most of these apps have access to virtually any food, including a surprising number of restaurant menus.

You might wonder, What if there's a restaurant or homecooked meal that I can't find in my nutrition app library? The answer is that you can usually find a very similar meal in your app that's close enough for tracking purposes. For instance, when you're at a backyard barbecue, the exact nutritional info for the ribs and coleslaw being served won't be in your food library. But there's almost always generic info for these types of foods—as well as restaurant versions of similar dishes—available in app libraries. In most cases, these options will be effective substitutes. On the rare occasions when you cannot find a close substitute, nearly all nutrition apps will allow you to manually enter new foods and meals. This is especially helpful at some restaurants, most of which now provide at least the caloric content of their meals right on their menus.

One very important component of logging and tracking your diet is being honest with yourself about portion sizes. When you're at home, measuring out portions and being exact is much easier. You can use measuring cups or a food scale to help with this. Gauging portion sizes is trickier when you're at a restaurant or social gathering. These situations require you to estimate, and unfortunately, people tend to underestimate their portions. While bringing measuring cups out with you in public isn't advisable, being conservative in your portion size estimations is a best practice. To ensure that you don't underestimate, logging a *higher* portion size than you think you've eaten is helpful. For instance, if you believe you ate one cup of potato salad, log a cup and a half; if you believe that you ate a four-ounce ice cream scoop, log a six-ounce scoop. While estimating portions isn't an exact science, it's a skill that improves with practice. If your weight goes up more than expected after a cheat meal, then you probably ate more than you estimated. When you get more skilled at estimating, you'll get surprisingly good at guessing what you'll weigh at your next morning weigh in.

Another benefit of logging all your meals in a nutrition app is that it can help keep the frequency of your deviations from a meal plan under control. Your food log should be used as an awareness tool to help better inform you when deviation is acceptable and when it's not. The secret to this is to check your log to see how you're tracking toward daily macros and calorie targets prior to eating anything. This behavior protocol is easy to implement with a nutrition app because you'll usually have your smart phone or device with you. While this strategy may sound simple, you'll be amazed at how a quick glance at your daily food log can significantly alter the decisions you make about food.

Memory is a terrible tool for keeping track of what you're eating. If you're not putting the information into an app, then you're probably uninformed about how you're tracking toward your goals at any given moment. In this uninformed state, we're more apt to make bad decisions about when deviation from a meal plan is okay. For instance, Nicole might think she stuck to her diet and wants to deviate during dinner, but she forgot about eating that free doughnut at the office that morning. Without an accurate meal log to check, she might proceed with her dinner plans, unaware that it would put her significantly over her calorie budget. Even though a single cheat meal probably won't have a significant impact, the real problem in this example is the decision-making *method*. Relying on memory to keep track of nutrition information leads to poor decision-making, and when this is done systematically, bad decisions become systemic.

If Nicole tracked what she ate with a nutrition app, she could check her log before deciding on dinner plans. This would remind her about the doughnut she'd eaten earlier and might sway her decisions about her next meal. She could decide to eat a lighter dinner to account for her earlier deviation (the morning doughnut). Or, she might decide to proceed with her dinner plans and then stick to her meal plan 100 percent for the rest of the week. The point is that checking her food log before making the choice allows her to better understand the potential outcome of either decision. This enables her to steer her fitness development in the desired direction. Making good decisions about when dietary deviation is acceptable is ultimately about your personal goals. Consistently checking your food log prior to eating gives you the opportunity to make the best decisions about diet and nutrition that align with your goals.

Cheat Days

At this point you're probably wondering, How much deviation from my core meal plan is acceptable? The answer is that it depends on how much friction you're willing to deal with and how fast you want to make progress. If you stick to your meal plan 100 percent of the time, you'll minimize friction and make progress at the fastest possible pace. Straying from this approach significantly increases the time and energy that's required to track your consumption and hit your nutritional targets. When you bring more friction into the process, you increase the likelihood that you'll lose track of your nutrition and stop making progress. In general, you should stick to your core meal plan 100 percent for most days of the week and allow yourself to deviate only on specific days—if at all.

Predesignating the days when you'll allow yourself to deviate from your core meals makes it easier to keep track of the consequences. You should predesignate the days you're most likely to deviate as your official "cheat days." For example, Lucas is more likely to stray from his core meal plan on Saturdays because that's when he spends time with family and friends. Knowing this, he allows himself a cheat day on Saturdays and sticks to his core meal plan the rest of the week. By predesignating when his cheat meals will be, he removes much of the uncertainty that comes with deciding when deviation from his plan is okay. This approach also removes much of the friction that comes from straying from a core meal plan haphazardly.

Dieting during Travel

Traveling can make it difficult to stick to a core meal plan. When you're away from home for multiple days, it can be tough not to deviate from what you normally eat. Most people experience this when they're away on vacation or a business trip. When traveling, you should consider where you'll be and what type of access you'll have to nutritious food. Maybe you'll be spending many days in airports or driving long distance. Regardless, the key is understanding the types of foods you'll have access to and taking time to build travel-specific meal plans that align with your goals. This requires doing research ahead of time to map out when and where the best opportunities are to find nutritious options.

For instance, you may have the opportunity to visit some great restaurants while traveling. If so, you can prescreen the menus and pick some options that will fit into your nutrition plan. Or perhaps you'll be frequenting a lot of convenience stores while on the road. In that case, you can generally find healthy options such as beef jerky, protein bars, and fruits. Identifying some staple foods that travel well is also helpful. You can prepack these foods and have healthy snack and meal options ready in the car or in a carry-on bag. The broad point with travel is that thinking ahead and building a plan will reduce the friction of trying to make healthy diet and nutrition choices in the moment.

When traveling, also consider the type of kitchen access you'll have once you arrive at wherever you're staying. If you have a full kitchen and a grocery store nearby, then you can probably stick to your normal core meal plan. Even if you don't have access to full kitchen amenities, you'll probably at least have a refrigerator and microwave. In these cases, you might have to make alterations to some of your core meals, but you can usually find viable substitutes for some of your staple foods. For instance, you might need to buy premade frozen hamburger patties instead of fresh ground beef. Or you might have to go with precooked frozen chicken breasts instead of fresh chicken. When it comes to travel, the meals and staple food options aren't always ideal, but you don't have to lose ground on your fitness goals if you think ahead and plan appropriately.

Conclusion

You are now equipped to use your new nutritional knowledge and dietary targets to build a core meal plan that's tailored to your fitness goals. You've also learned effective methods for tracking what you eat and how to use that information to systematically make the best dieting decisions possible. As you implement these strategies and tactics, remember that the key to diet and nutrition is knowing your goals and grasping how your behaviors can impact attaining them. The system laid out in chapters 12–14 provides the most efficient path to developing good diet and nutrition habits. Creating these healthy habits will reduce the friction involved with making good diet and nutritional decisions. This will provide you with the best chance of sticking to your core meal plan and make the pursuit of your fitness goals as easy as possible.

Conclusion

IN THIS BOOK, YOU HAVE learned that most people's challenge with getting and staying fit is a failure to develop fitness-promoting habits that mesh with their daily routines. You now understand that most of today's popular fitness solutions—exercise and nutrition—don't prioritize building sustainable habits, which makes them incompatible with the way most people live. You have learned to develop effective habits using a fully integrated system of strategies, tactics, and tools that eliminate friction from diet and exercise, which will allow you to attain and sustain your fitness goals. You now understand that by minimizing the friction that often comes with diet and exercise, you make it possible to overcome the two most prevalent factors that prevent most people from getting and staying fit: lack of time and energy.

Now you should take action! As you begin implementing what you've learned in this book, remember that the methods are not a two-week crash diet or a shortcut program for building muscles; they're part of a fitness system designed for people who've realized that they have only one life to live and want it to be the best life possible. The life-enhancing philosophy, strategies, tactics, and tools will all work together to help you develop sustainable habits that will last a lifetime. If you can't implement everything I've suggested simultaneously, implement the parts that fit into your life most easily. Once these initial pieces become habits, you can come back later and implement the system more fully. By implementing my methods, you will eliminate the friction that normally comes with diet and exercise, maximize the use of your time and energy, and achieve your fitness goals!

After your first reading, let this book continue to be your roadmap and reference guide along the way. You won't always remember all the necessary details, so reread it when you need a refresher. Though new scientific advances are often made in the exercise and nutrition fields, this system was built on fundamental principles that will stand the test of time. Go forth with confidence and count on *The Friction Factor* system to guide your lifelong journey toward healthier and happier living.

Notes

Introduction

1. Diane Thieke, "Out of Shape? Americans Turn to Exercise to Get Fit," ReportLinker, May 31, 2017, https://www.reportlinker.com/insight /shape-americans-exercise-get-fit.html; Paul D. Loprinzi et al., "Healthy Lifestyle Characteristics and Their Joint Association with Cardiovascular Disease Biomarkers in US Adults," *Mayo Clinic Proceedings* 91, no. 4 (April 2016): 432–442, https://doi.org/10.1016/j.mayocp.2016.01.009.

2. Ellie, "60 percent of Americans Plan to Get in Shape in 2019," *Freeletics* (blog), 2019, https://www.freeletics.com/en/blog/posts/the -freeletics-dare-to-be-free-survey/.

3. IFIC Foundation, "2012 Food and Health Survey," Food Insight, April 1, 2012, https://foodinsight.org/2012-food-and-health-survey/.

Chapter 2

1. Joseph Luciani, "Why 80 Percent of New Year's Resolutions Fail," *U.S. News & World Report*, December 29, 2015, https://health.usnews.com /health-news/blogs/eat-run/articles/2015-12-29/why-80-percent-of-new -years-resolutions-fail.

2. Gryphon Adams, "Is It Good to Exercise Every Day for Weight Loss?," Livestrong.com, accessed April 25, 2021, https://www.livestrong.com/article /407045-is-it-good-to-exercise-every-day-if-im-trying-to-lose-weight/ (site discontinued); "NWCR Facts," National Weight Control Registry, accessed April 25, 2021, http://www.nwcr.ws/Research/default.htm.

3. Debra Fulghum Bruce, "Exercise and Depression: Endorphins, Reducing Stress, and More," WebMD, February 18, 2020, https://www .webmd.com/depression/guide/exercise-depression.

4. Bruce, "Exercise and Depression"; Jennifer Berry, "Endorphins: Effects and How to Increase Levels," *Medical News Today*, February 6, 2018, https://www.medicalnewstoday.com/articles/320839; Emily Laurence, "Endorphins and Exercise: How Intense Does a Workout Have to Be for the 'High' to Kick in?," Well+Good, July 27, 2018, https://www.wellandgood .com/endorphins-and-exercise/.

5. Jane Porter, "How Exercise Changes Your Brain To Be Better at Basically Everything," *Fast Company*, November 3, 2014, https://www .fastcompany.com/3037894/how-exercise-changes-your-brain-to-be -better-at-basically-everything; Ben Martynoga, "How Physical Exercise Makes Your Brain Work Better," *Guardian*, June 18, 2016, https://www .theguardian.com/education/2016/jun/18/how-physical-exercise-makes -your-brain-work-better.

6. Colette Bouchez, "Exercise for Energy: Workouts That Work," WebMD, August 7, 2009, https://www.webmd.com/fitness-exercise/features /exercise-for-energy-workouts-that-work.

7. "Exercising for Better Sleep," Johns Hopkins Medicine, accessed April 25, 2021, https://www.hopkinsmedicine.org/health/wellness-and -prevention/exercising-for-better-sleep.

8. "Exercise Suppresses Appetite by Affecting Appetite Hormones," *ScienceDaily*, December 19, 2008, https://www.sciencedaily.com /releases/2008/12/081211081446.htm; David R. Broom et al., "Influence of Resistance and Aerobic Exercise on Hunger, Circulating Levels of Acylated Ghrelin, and Peptide YY in Healthy Males," *American Journal of Physiol- ogy—Regulatory, Integrative and Comparative Physiology* 296, no. 1 (January 2009): 33, https://doi.org/10.1152/ajpregu.90706.2008; Efthimia Karra, Keval Chandarana, and Rachel L. Batterham, "The Role of Peptide YY in Appetite Regulation and Obesity," *Journal of Physiology* 587, no. 1 (January 2009): 19, https://doi.org/10.1113/jphysiol.2008.164269; Elaine Iandoli, "Research Explains Link between Exercise and Appetite Loss," Albert Einstein College of Medicine, April 24, 2018, http://einsteinmed.edu/news /releases/1296/research-explains-link-between-exercise-and-appetite-loss/.

9. *McGraw-Hill Concise Dictionary of Modern Medicine*, s.v. "overtrain- ing," accessed April 25, 2021, https://medical-dictionary.thefreedictionary .com/overtraining.

10. Damon L. Swift et al., "The Role of Exercise and Physical Activity in Weight Loss and Maintenance," *Progress in Cardiovascular Diseases* 56, no. 4 (January–February 2014): 8, accessed April 30, 2021, https://doi .org/10.1016/j.pcad.2013.09.012; Luke Carlson et al., "Neither Repetition Duration nor Number of Muscle Actions Affect Strength Increases, Body Composition, Muscle Size, or Fasted Blood Glucose in Trained Males and Females," *Applied Physiology, Nutrition, and Metabolism* 44, no. 2 (February 2019): 1, https://doi.org/10.1139/apnm-2018-0376.

11. James Clear, "How Long Does It Actually Take to Form a New Habit, (Backed by Science)," *HuffPost*, June 10, 2014, https://www.huffpost.com /entry/forming-new-habits_b_5104807; Phillippa Lally et al., "How Are Habits Formed: Modelling Habit Formation in the Real World," *European Journal of Social Psychology* 40, no. 6 (July 2009): 998–1009, https://doi.org /10.1002/ejsp.674.

Chapter 3

1. *Random House Kernerman Webster's College Dictionary*, s.v. "motivation," accessed May 1, 2021, https://www.thefreedictionary.com/motivation.

2. Ellen Gans, "How to Choose the Best Gym Membership—Costs & Ways to Save," Money Crashers, June 10, 2015, https://www.moneycrashers .com/choose-best-gym-membership-costs/.

Chapter 4

1. Stacey Colino, "The Hazards of Decision Overload," *U.S. News & World Report*, March 2015, 2017, https://health.usnews.com/wellness/mind /articles/2017-03-15/the-hazards-of-decision-overload; John Tierney, "Do You Suffer from Decision Fatigue?," *New York Times*, https://www.nytimes .com/2011/08/21/magazine/do-you-suffer-from-decision-fatigue.html.

2. Brian Tracy, *Eat That Frog!: 21 Great Ways to Stop Procrastinating and Get More Done in Less Time* (San Francisco: Berrett-Koehler, 2007).

3. Jeffrey M. Jones, "In U.S., 40 Percent Get Less Than Recommended Amount of Sleep," Gallup, December 19, 2013, https://news.gallup.com /poll/166553/less-recommended-amount-sleep.aspx; "Sleep and Sleep Disorders: Data and Statistics," Centers for Disease Control and Prevention,

May 2, 2017, https://www.cdc.gov/sleep/data_statistics.html; Jennifer Casarella, "Tips to Reduce Stress and Sleep Better," WebMD, December 14, 2019, https://www.webmd.com/sleep-disorders/tips-reduce-stress.

4. "Twelve Simple Tips to Improve Your Sleep," Division of Sleep Medicine at Harvard Medical School, December 18, 2007, http://healthysleep.med.harvard.edu/healthy/getting/overcoming/tips.

5. Amanda MacMillan, "20 Things You Shouldn't Do Before Bed," Health.com, April 8, 2015, http://www.health.com/mind-body/20-things-you-shouldn-t-do-before-bed.

6. "How Technology Impacts Sleep Quality," Sleep.org, March 12, 2021, https://www.sleep.org/ways-technology-affects-sleep/; Gianluca Tosini, Ian Ferguson, and Kazuo Tsubota, "Effects of Blue Light on the Circadian System and Eye Physiology," *Molecular Vision* 22 (January 2016): 61–72, https://www.ncbi.nlm.nih.gov/pmc/articles/PMC4734149/; Leena Tähkämö, Timo Partonen, and Anu-Katriina Pesonen, "Systematic Review of Light Exposure Impact on Human Circadian Rhythm," *Chronobiology International* 36, no. 2 (October 2018): 151–170, https://doi.org/10.1080/07420528.2018.1527773.

7. "What Is the Best Temperature for Sleep?," Sleep.org, March 12, 2021, https://www.sleep.org/temperature-for-sleep/; Kazue Okamoto-Mizuno and Koh Mizuno, "Effects of Thermal Environment on Sleep and Circadian Rhythm," *Journal of Physiological Anthropology* 31, no.1 (May 2012): 14, https://doi.org/10.1186/1880-6805-31-14; Edward C. Harding, Nicholas P. Franks, and William Wisden, "The Temperature Dependence of Sleep," *Frontiers in Neuroscience* 13 (April 2019): 336, https://doi.org/10.3389/fnins.2019.00336.

8. MacMillan, "20 Things"; Christy L. Hoffman, Matthew Browne, and Bradley P. Smith, "Human-Animal Co-Sleeping: An Actigraphy-Based Assessment of Dogs' Impacts on Women's Nighttime Movements," *Animals* 10, no. 2 (February 2020): 278, https://doi.org/10.3390/ani10020278.

Chapter 5

1. Chris Iliades, "What Counts as Aerobic Exercise? Here's Everything You Need to Know about How to Get the Cardio You Need," Everyday Health, July 6, 2021, https://www.everydayhealth.com/fitness/workouts/why-you-need-aerobic-exercise.aspx.

2. "American Heart Association Recommendations for Physical Activity in Adults and Kids," American Heart Association, April 18, 2018, https://www.heart.org/en/healthy-living/fitness/fitness-basics/aha-recs-for-physical-activity-in-adults.

3. Erin Kelly, "What You Need to Know About Anaerobic Exercise," *Healthline*, March 6, 2019, https://www.healthline.com/health/fitness-exercise/anaerobic-exercise; Laura Dolson, "The Role of Glycogen in Diet and Exercise," *Verywell Fit*, July 17, 2019, https://www.verywellfit.com/what-is-glycogen-2242008.

4. Jen Mueller and Nicole Nichols, "Reference Guide to Anaerobic Exercise," *SparkPeople*, February 27, 2008, https://www.sparkpeople.com/resource/fitness_articles.asp?id=1035; "The Benefits of Anaerobic Exercise," Piedmont Healthcare, accessed May 2, 2021, https://www.piedmont.org/living-better/the-benefits-of-anaerobic-exercise.

5. "Want to Live Longer and Better? Do Strength Training," *Harvard Health*, February 15, 2021, https://www.health.harvard.edu/staying-healthy/want-to-live-longer-and-better-do-strength-training.

6. Brad J. Schoenfeld, "The Mechanisms of Muscle Hypertrophy and Their Application to Resistance Training," *Journal of Strength and Conditioning Research* 24, no. 10 (October 2010): 2857–2858, https://doi.org/10.1519/jsc.0b013e3181e840f3.

7. Monika Guszkowska, "Effects of Exercise on Anxiety, Depression and Mood," *Psychiatria Polska* 38, no. 4 (July–August 2004): 611–620, https://pubmed.ncbi.nlm.nih.gov/15518309/; Sarah Elizabeth Richards, "7 Benefits of Strength Training That Go beyond Building Muscle," *NBCNews.com*, February 9, 2018, https://www.nbcnews.com/better/health/7-benefits-strength-training-go-way-beyond-building-muscle-ncna845936.

8. Fiataraone Singh et al., "ACSM Guidelines for Strength Training: Featured Download," American College of Sports Medicine, July 31, 2019, https://www.acsm.org/blog-detail/acsm-certified-blog/2019/07/31/acsm-guidelines-for-strength-training-featured-download.

9. Sabrena Jo et al., eds., *The Exercise Professional's Guide to Personal Training* (San Diego: American Council on Exercise, 2020), 231.

10. Kristeen Cherney, "How Accurate Are Body Fat Scales?," *Healthline*, July 22, 2019, https://www.healthline.com/health/body-fat-scale-accuracy.

11. Corin B. Arenas, "Fat Free Mass Index: Importance and Maintaining the Right Levels," Calculators.org, October 12, 2019, https://www.calculators.org/health/ffmi.php.

12. Joel Hoekstra, "How Much of Your Body Mass Is Actually Muscle—and How Do You Measure It?," Livestrong.com, February 21, 2020, https://www.livestrong.com/article/462608-how-much-of-your-body-mass-is-actually-muscle/.

13. "Percent Body Fat Norms for Men and Women," American Council on Exercise, accessed May 4, 2021, https://www.acefitness.org/education-and-resources/lifestyle/tools-calculators/percent-body-fat-calculator/.

14. "ACSM's Guidelines for Exercise Testing and Prescription," American College of Sports Medicine, 2019, https://www.acsm.org/docs/default-source/publications-files/getp10_tables-4-4-4-5-updated.pdf.

15. "Helpful Formulas," American Council on Exercise, February 20, 2022, https://www.acefitness.org/ptresources/pdfs/Formulas.pdf.

Chapter 6

1. Damon L. Swift et al., "The Role of Exercise and Physical Activity in Weight Loss and Maintenance," *Progress in Cardiovascular Diseases* 56, no. 4 (January–February 2014): 8, https://doi.org/10.1016/j.pcad.2013.09.012; Luke Carlson et al., "Neither Repetition Duration nor Number of Muscle Actions Affect Strength Increases, Body Composition, Muscle Size, or Fasted Blood Glucose in Trained Males and Females," *Applied Physiology, Nutrition, and Metabolism* 44, no. 2 (February 2019): 1, https://doi.org/10.1139/apnm-2018-0376.

2. "Losing Weight," Centers for Disease Control and Prevention, August 17, 2020, https://www.cdc.gov/healthyweight/losing_weight/index.html; Mayo Clinic Staff "Weight Loss: 6 Strategies for Success," Mayo Clinic, December 18, 2019, https://www.mayoclinic.org/healthy-lifestyle/weight-loss/in-depth/weight-loss/art-20047752; Ryan Raman, "Is It Bad to Lose Weight Too Quickly?," *Healthline*, October 29, 2017, https://www.healthline.com/nutrition/losing-weight-too-fast; Roel G. Vink et al., "The Effect of Rate of Weight Loss on Long Term Weight Regain in Adults with Overweight and Obesity," *Obesity* 24, no. 2 (February 2016): 326, https://doi.org/10.1002/oby.21346; "Gallstones," National Institute of Diabetes and

Digestive and Kidney Diseases, accessed May 10, 2021, https://www.niddk
.nih.gov/health-information/digestive-diseases/gallstones.

3. Jane Chertoff, "Muscular Hypertrophy and Your Workout," *Health-line*, February 26, 2019, https://www.healthline.com/health/muscular
-hypertrophy.

4. A. M. Pearson, "Muscle Growth and Exercise," *Critical Reviews in Food Science and Nutrition* 29, no. 3 (1990), https://doi.org/10.1080
/10408399009527522; Natalie Digate Muth, "What Are the Guidelines for Percentage of Body Fat Loss?," American Council on Exercise, December 2, 2009, https://www.acefitness.org/education-and-resources/lifestyle
/blog/112/what-are-the-guidelines-for-percentage-of-body-fat-loss/.

5. Muth, "Guidelines for Percentage,"; Amy J. Hector et al., "Pronounced Energy Restriction with Elevated Protein Intake Results in No Change in Proteolysis and Reductions in Skeletal Muscle Protein Synthesis That Are Mitigated by Resistance Exercise," *FASEB Journal* 32, no. 1 (January 2018): 274, https://doi.org/10.1096/fj.201700158RR; Amely M. Verreijen et al., "Effect of a High Protein Diet and/or Resistance Exercise on the Preservation of Fat Free Mass during Weight Loss in Overweight and Obese Older Adults: A Randomized Controlled Trial," *Nutrition Journal* 16, no. 10 (February 2017): 7, https://doi.org/10.1186/s12937-017-0229-6; Adam Tzur, "Gaining Muscle Mass in a Deficit vs. Bulking (Research Review)," Sci-Fit, April 25, 2018, https://sci-fit.net/bulking-deficit-gaining/.

6. Jay Blahnik, "How Much Muscle Can You Gain & How Fast Can You Build It?," Workout Routine, July 24, 2020, https://www.aworkoutroutine.com/how-much-muscle-can-you-gain/; Erin Nitschke, "How Muscle Grows," American Council on Exercise, August 30, 2017, https://www
.acefitness.org/education-and-resources/lifestyle/blog/6538/how-muscle
-grows/; Chelsea Ritschel, "This Is How Much Muscle You Can Gain in a Month, According to Experts," *Independent*, March 5, 2021, https://www
.independent.co.uk/life-style/health-and-families/muscle-gain-fast-body
-fat-loss-b1775326.html.

7. Nitschke, "How Muscle."

8. Jessie Newell, "The Basics of Exercise Science (Part 5)," American Council on Exercise, April 10, 2015, https://www.acefitness.org/fitness
-certifications/ace-answers/exam-preparation-blog/5371/the-basics-of
-exercise-science-part-5/; "Why It Becomes Harder to Build Muscle Over

Time," Cathe, accessed May 13, 2021, https://cathe.com/why-it-becomes
-harder-to-build-muscle-over-time/.

9. Paul Saenger, "Dose Effects of Growth Hormone during Puberty,"
Hormone Research 60, no. 1 (2003): 52, https://doi.org/10.1159/000071226;
Emily Cronkleton, "Side Effects of HGH: What You Should Know,"
Healthline, March 29, 2019, https://www.healthline.com/health/hgh-side
-effects; "Physical Changes during Puberty," healthychildren.org, December
19, 2014, https://www.healthychildren.org/English/ages-stages/gradeschool
/puberty/Pages/Physical-Development-of-School-Age-Children.aspx.

10. Matt Danielsson, "The Myth of Turning Fat into Muscle," Body
-building.com, April 19, 2018, https://www.bodybuilding.com/content/the
-myth-of-turning-fat-into-muscle.html.

11. "Sports and Exercise among Americans," US Bureau of Labor Statistics, August 04, 2016, accessed May 15, 2021, https://www.bls.gov/opub
/ted/2016/sports-and-exercise-among-americans.htm.

12. Brian Alexander, "Ideal to Real: What the 'Perfect' Body Really Looks
Like for Men and Women," *Today*, June 23, 2016, https://www.today.com
/health/ideal-real-what-perfect-body-really-looks-men-women-t83731;
Kara L. Crossley, Piers L. Cornelissen, and Martin J. Tovee, "What Is an
Attractive Body? Using an Interactive 3D Program to Create the Ideal Body
for You and Your Partner," *PLOS ONE* 7, no. 11 (November 2012): 8–9,
https://doi.org/10.1371/journal.pone.0050601; Jessica Salvatore and Jeanne
Marecek, "Gender in the Gym: Evaluation Concerns as Barriers to Women's
Weight Lifting," *Sex Roles* 63, no. 7 (October 2010): 6, http://dx.doi.org
/10.1007/s11199-010-9800-8.

13. Salvatore and Marecek, "Gender," 6, 8–11.

14. Salvatore and Marecek, "Gender," 6.

15. *Physical Activity Guidelines for Americans*, 2nd ed. United States
Department of Health and Human Services (Washington, DC : US Department of Health and Human Services, 2018), https://health.gov/sites
/default/files/2019-09/Physical_Activity_Guidelines_2nd_edition.pdf;
Caroline Wilbert, "Strength Training Is Good for Seniors," WebMD, July 8,
2009, https://www.webmd.com/healthy-aging/news/20090708
/strength-training-is-good-for-seniors.

Chapter 8

1. "Progression Models in Resistance Training for Healthy Adults," *Medicine & Science in Sports & Exercise* 41, no. 3 (March 2009): 691, http://dx.doi.org/10.1249/MSS.0b013e3181915670.

2. Conor Heffernan, "An Early History of Weightlifting," Physical Culture Study, November 18, 2014, https://physicalculturestudy.com/2014/11/18/an-early-history-of-weightlifting/.

3. Ryan Patrick, "6 Compound Training Movements Build Serious Mass!" Bodybuilding.com, April 1, 2020, https://www.bodybuilding.com/content/6-compound-movements-build-mass.html.

4. Patrick, "6 Compound"; Jay Blahnik, "Movement Patterns: Exercises for Horizontal & Vertical Push & Pull, Quad & Hip Dominant, and More," Workout Routine, January 20, 2018, https://www.aworkoutroutine.com/movement-patterns/.

5. Patrick, "6 Compound,"; Kevin Rail, "What Muscle Group Do Cable Rows Work?," Livestrong.com, accessed May 16, 2021, https://www.livestrong.com/article/537832-what-muscle-group-do-cable-rows-work/; Blahnik, "Movement Patterns."

6. Henry Halse, "Muscles Used in a Military Press," Livestrong.com, accessed May 16, 2021, https://www.livestrong.com/article/294070-muscles-used-in-a-military-press/; Blahnik, "Movement Patterns."

7. Patrick, "6 Compound," Blahnik, "Movement Patterns."

8. "Pull-Ups," American Council on Exercise, accessed May 16, 2021, https://www.acefitness.org/education-and-resources/lifestyle/exercise-library/191/pull-ups/.

9. Patrick, "6 Compound."

10. Riana Rohmann, "Mastering the Deadlift," American Council on Exercise, October 30, 2013, https://www.acefitness.org/education-and-resources/lifestyle/blog/3584/mastering-the-deadlift/.

11. Patrick, "6 Compound."

12. Franklin Antoian, "5 Lunge Variations You Need to Try," American Council on Exercise, February 15, 2016, https://www.acefitness.org/education-and-resources/professional/expert-articles/5818/5-lunge-variations-you-need-to-try/.

13. Stanley P. Brown, *Introduction to Exercise Science* (Baltimore: Lippincott Williams & Wilkins, 2001), 280–281.

Chapter 9

1. Edward Stenger et al., "Abs! Abs! Abs!," American Council on Exercise, April 2014, https://www.acefitness.org/education-and-resources /professional/prosource/april-2014/3764/abs-abs-abs/.

2. "Crunch," American Council on Exercise, accessed May 23, 2021, https://www.acefitness.org/education-and-resources/lifestyle/exercise -library/52/crunch/.

3. "Are Squats and Deadlifts Enough for Your Ab Definition?," Cathe, accessed May 23, 2021, https://cathe.com/are-squats-and-deadlifts-enough -for-your-ab-definition.

4. Stenger, "Abs! Abs! Abs."

5. "Target Heart Rates Chart," American Heart Association, March 9, 2021, https://www.heart.org/en/healthy-living/fitness/fitness-basics/target -heart-rates.

6. Sabrena Jo et al., eds., *The Exercise Professional's Guide to Personal Training* (San Diego: American Council on Exercise, 2020), 280.

7. Jo et al., *Exercise Professional's Guide,* 155–158.

8. Emily Cronkleton, "Is Running in Place a Good Workout?," *Healthline*, March 30, 2020, https://www.healthline.com/health/fitness-exercise /running-in-place.

9. Ashley Marcin, "Benefits of Jumping Jacks and How to Do Them," *Healthline*, May 23, 2018, https://www.healthline.com/health/fitness -exercise/jumping-jacks.

10. Leanna Skarnulis, "Skipping Rope Doesn't Skip Workout," WebMD, accessed March 3, 2022, https://www.webmd.com/fitness-exercise/features /skipping-rope-doesnt-skip-workout.

11. Jo et al., *Exercise Professional's Guide*, 690.

Chapter 10

1. Fiatarone Singh et al., "ACSM Guidelines for Strength Training: Featured Download," American College of Sports Medicine, July 31, 2019, https://www.acsm.org/blog-detail/acsm-certified-blog/2019/07/31/acsm -guidelines-for-strength-training-featured-download.

2. Pete McCall, "7 Benefits of Sleep for Exercise Recovery," American Council on Exercise, Mach 11, 2021, https://www.acefitness.org/education

-and-resources/lifestyle/blog/7818/7-benefits-of-sleep-for-exercise
-recovery/.

3. Michael Berg and Brad Schoenfeld, "How Many Reps Will Build the Most Muscle?," *Men's Journal*, May 22, 2020, https://www.mensjournal.com /health-fitness/rep-range-builds-most-muscle/.

4. Berg and Schoenfeld, "How Many Reps"; Jane Chertoff, "Muscular Hypertrophy and Your Workout," *Healthline*, February 26, 2019, https:// www.healthline.com/health/muscular-hypertrophy; Brad J. Schoenfeld, "The Mechanisms of Muscle Hypertrophy and Their Application to Resistance Training," *Journal of Strength and Conditioning Research* 24, no. 10 (October 2010): 2867, http://dx.doi.org/10.1519/JSC.0b013e3181e840f3.

5. Berg and Schoenfeld, "How Many Reps"; Jonathan W. Evans, "Periodized Resistance Training for Enhancing Skeletal Muscle Hypertrophy and Strength: A Mini-Review," *Frontiers in Physiology* 10, (January 2019): 5, https://doi.org/10.3389/fphys.2019.00013.

6. Evans, "Periodized Resistance."

Chapter 11

1. "Strength Training 101," American Council on Exercise, January 29, 2009, https://www.acefitness.org/education-and-resources/lifestyle/blog /6695/strength-training-101/.

2. Bill Hartman, "How Long Should I Rest between Sets to Build Muscle?," *Men's Health*, November 7, 2011, https://www.menshealth.com/fitness /a19540335/how-long-should-i-rest-between-sets-to-build-muscle/.

3. Hartman, "How Long."

4. Hartman, "How Long."

5. Mayo Clinic Staff, "Rev up Your Workout with Interval Training," Mayo Clinic, June 23, 2020, https://www.mayoclinic.org/healthy-lifestyle /fitness/in-depth/interval-training/art-20044588.

6. Daniel J. Green, "ACE-Sponsored Research: Is HIIT Resistance Exercise Superior to Traditional Resistance Training?," American Council on Exercise, June 2018, https://www.acefitness.org/education-and-resources /professional/certified/june-2018/7011/ace-sponsored-research-is-hiit -resistance-exercise-superior-to-traditional-resistance-training/.

7. "Interval Training," American Council on Exercise, January 8, 2009, https://www.acefitness.org/education-and-resources/lifestyle/blog/6615/interval-training/.

8. Jenessa Connor, "How Much Cardio Do You Really Need?," *Men's Journal*, March 30, 2018, https://www.mensjournal.com/health-fitness/how-much-cardio-do-you-really-need-w488887/; Jonathan Ross, "Why We Still Need Cardio Training: A More Effective Approach," American Council on Exercise, March 9, 2015, https://www.acefitness.org/education-and-resources/professional/expert-articles/5330/why-we-still-need-cardio-training-a-more-effective-approach/.

9. Mayo Clinic Staff, "Exercise Intensity: How to Measure It," Mayo Clinic, August 6, 2019, https://www.mayoclinic.org/healthy-lifestyle/fitness/in-depth/exercise-intensity/art-20046887.

10. Connor, "How Much."

11. Mayo, "Exercise Intensity."

12. Mayo, "Exercise Intensity."

13. Sabrena Jo et al., eds., *The Exercise Professional's Guide to Personal Training* (San Diego: American Council on Exercise, 2020), 383.

14. Jo et al., *Exercise Professional's Guide*, 382.

15. Jo et al., *Exercise Professional's Guide*, 383.

Chapter 12

1. "Benefits of Protein," WebMD, October 12, 2020, https://www.webmd.com/diet/benefits-protein1; "Proteins: Building Blocks of the Body," Otsuka Pharmaceutical, accessed May 6, 2021, https://www.otsuka.co.jp/en/nutraceutical/about/nutrition/sports-nutrition/essential-nutrients/proteins.html; "What Are Proteins and What Do They Do?," Medline Plus, *US National Library of Medicine*, August 4, 2020, https://medlineplus.gov/genetics/understanding/howgeneswork/protein/; "Amino Acids," Medline Plus, *US National Library of Medicine*, July 2, 2020, https://medlineplus.gov/ency/article/002222.htm; Emily Cronkleton, "Are There Risks Associated with Eating Too Much Protein?," *Healthline*, April 13, 2020, https://www.healthline.com/health/too-much-protein.

2. "Protein," Better Health Channel, March 12, 2020, https://www.betterhealth.vic.gov.au/health/healthyliving/protein.

3. US Department of Agriculture and US Department of Health and Human Services, *Dietary Guidelines for Americans, 2020-2025*, 9th edition (December 2020), 133, https://www.dietaryguidelines.gov/sites/default/files/2020-12/Dietary_Guidelines_for_Americans_2020-2025.pdf.

4. Sabrenda Jo et al., eds., *The Exercise Professional's Guide to Personal Training* (San Diego: American Council on Exercise, 2020), 563.

5. Brad Schoenfeld, *Science and Development of Muscle Hypertrophy*, 2nd edition (Champaign: Human Kinetics, 2021), 215–217.

6. "Carbohydrates," Medline Plus, *US National Library of Medicine*, July 1, 2020, https://medlineplus.gov/carbohydrates.html; Kristeen Cherney, "Simple Carbohydrates vs. Complex Carbohydrates," *Healthline*, June 20, 2020, https://www.healthline.com/health/food-nutrition/simple-carbohy-drates-complex-carbohydrates; "How Sugar Converts to Fat," University of Utah Health, August 22, 2018, https://healthcare.utah.edu/the-scope/shows.php?shows=0_7frg4jjd.

7. Cherney, "Simple Carbohydrates"; "Simple Carbohydrates," Medline Plus, *US National Library of Medicine*, January 26, 2020, https://medlineplus.gov/ency/imagepages/19534.htm; "Carbohydrates," *American Heart Association*, April 16, 2018, https://www.heart.org/en/healthy-living/healthy-eating/eat-smart/nutrition-basics/carbohydrates.

8. *Recommended Dietary Allowances*, 10th ed., (Washington, DC: National Academy Press, 1989), https://www.ncbi.nlm.nih.gov/books/NBK234933/; Cherney, "Simple Carbohydrates."; "Complex Carbohy-drates," Medline Plus, *US National Library of Medicine*, February 22, 2018, https://medlineplus.gov/ency/imagepages/19529.htm; Mayo Clinic Staff, "Dietary Fiber: Essential for a Healthy Diet," Mayo Clinic, November 16, 2018, https://www.mayoclinic.org/healthy-lifestyle/nutrition-and-healthy-eating/in-depth/fiber/art-20043983.

9. US Department of Agriculture and US Department of Health and Human Services, *Dietary Guidelines for Americans, 2020-2025*, 133.

10. Brad Schoenfeld, *Science and Development of Muscle Hypertrophy Second Edition* (Champaign: Human Kinetics, 2021), 217-220.

11. "Dietary Fats Explained," Medline Plus, *US National Library of Medi-cine*, July 13, 202020, https://medlineplus.gov/ency/patientinstructions/000104.htm.

12. Mayo Clinic Staff, "Dietary Fat: Know Which to Choose," Mayo Clinic, February 1, 2019, https://www.mayoclinic.org/healthy-lifestyle /nutrition-and-healthy-eating/in-depth/fat/art-20045550; "Facts about Saturated Fats," Medline Plus, *US National Library of Medicine*, April 23, 2018, https://medlineplus.gov/ency/patientinstructions/000838.htm; "Facts about Trans Fats," Medline Plus, *US National Library of Medicine*, April 23, 2018, https://medlineplus.gov/ency/patientinstructions/000786 .htm.

13. "The Truth about Fats: The Good, the Bad, and the In-between," *Harvard Health*, December 11, 2019, https://www.health.harvard.edu /staying-healthy/the-truth-about-fats-bad-and-good.

14. US Department of Agriculture and US Department of Health and Human Services, *Dietary Guidelines*, 133.

15. Schoenfeld, *Science and Development*, 221–222.

16. "Water in Diet," Medline Plus, *US National Library of Medicine*, July 3, 2019, https://medlineplus.gov/ency/article/002471.htm; "Functions of Water in the Body," Mayo Clinic, accessed August 10, 2020, https://www. mayoclinic.org/healthy-lifestyle/nutrition-and-healthy-eating/multimedia /functions-of-water-in-the-body/img-20005799; "7 Reasons Why Body-builders Need More Water," Bodybuilding.com, February 25, 2019, https:// www.bodybuilding.com/fun/animalpak21.htm; Jennifer Soong, "What Counts as Water? Stay Hydrated and Healthy," WebMD, September 9, 2011, https://www.webmd.com/parenting/features/healthy-beverages.

17. Kris Gunnars, "How Much Water Should You Drink Per Day?," Healthline, April 21, 2020, https://www.healthline.com/nutrition/how -much-water-should-you-drink-per-day; Barbara Gordon, "How Much Water Do You Need," *Eat Right Academy of Nutrition and Dietetics*, November 6, 2019, https://www.eatright.org/food/nutrition/healthy-eating/how -much-water-do-you-need.

18. Soong, "What Counts."

19. Soong, "What Counts."

20. Lizzie Streit, "Micronutrients: Types, Functions, Benefits and More," *Healthline*, September 27, 2018, https://www.healthline.com/nutrition /micronutrients.

21. "Losing Weight," Centers for Disease Control and Prevention, February 4, 2020, https://www.cdc.gov/healthyweight/losing_weight/index

.html; "Weight Loss: 6 Strategies for Success," Mayo Clinic, December 18, 2019, https://www.mayoclinic.org/healthy-lifestyle/weight-loss/in-depth /weight-loss/art-20047752. "How to Gain Healthy Weight," *Sanford Health News*, January 18, 2019, https://news.sanfordhealth.org/sports-medicine /weight-gain-performance/.

Chapter 13

1. US Department of Agriculture and US Department of Health and Human Services, *Dietary Guidelines*, 18.

2. Natalie Digate Muth et al., eds., *The Exercise Professional's Guide to Personal Training* (San Diego: American Council on Exercise, 2020), 174–175.

Index

ab exercises, 150–155
aerobic exercise. *See* cardio exercise
alarm clocks, 67–68
American College of Sports Medicine, 77
American Council on Exercise, 151
American Heart Association, 75
amino acids, 202
anaerobic exercise. *See* strength-training exercises
anchoring, 50–51

barbell exercises
    back extension, 144
    bench press, 120–123
    dead lift, 137–138, 141–142
batch cooking, 222–223, 228–229
Baumeister, Roy, 58
bedtime routine, 61–66
bench press, 120–123
BMI (body mass index), 80
body composition
    daily tracking of, 105–113
    definition of, 77
    measuring, 77–83
    setting goals for, 77, 84–89, 90, 92

body fat
    calories and, 93
    converting into muscle, myth of, 99–100
    muscle mass and, 92
    reducing, 93–94
body-fat percentage
    age-based guidelines for, 85
    changes in, 106–109, 111
    daily tracking of, 106
    measuring, 78–79
    norms for, 80
    setting target for, 84–86, 92
body types, "ideal," 101–103
body weight
    daily tracking of, 105–106
    measuring, 78
    setting target for, 86–87, 92
    See also weight gain; weight loss
breakfast
    considerations for, 230
    examples of, 239, 244, 246
bulking-up myth, 100–101

caffeinated drinks, 208
calipers, 78–79

calorie deficit, 93–94
calorie-efficient foods, 218–219
calories
    burning, 30, 74, 93–94
    calculating target for, 211, 213
    definition of, 93
    empty, 204
    of macronutrients, 210
    per-meal targets for, 231–233
    traditional approach to counting,
        215–216, 251
calorie surplus, 93
carbohydrates (carbs)
    complex, 204–205, 225
    muscle development and, 205
    per-meal targets for, 231–233
    prep time and, 228–229
    processed foods and, 225
    recommended daily allowance
        (RDA) for, 205
    role of, 204
    simple, 204
    sources of, 204–205, 226–227
    staples, 225–229
cardio exercise (aerobic exercise)
    benefits of, 74
    burning calories and, 74, 93–94
    definition of, 74
    examples of, 74
    goal for, 75, 89
    heart rate and, 155–156, 159
    interval training and, 186–187
    options for, 156–159
CDC (Centers for Disease Control
    and Prevention), 61, 189
change, possibility of, 1
cheat meals/days, 249–250, 254–255
chin-ups, 131–135
cholesterol, 206

circuit training, 187
clocks, 67–68
coffee, 208
complex carbohydrates, 204–205
complexity, as enemy of success, 4,
    216
compound exercises, 118–120,
    150
cooking, 222–223, 228–229
cool-downs, 193, 194
core daily meals
    benefits of, 216–217
    building, 229, 235–237, 241
    examples of, 238–240, 244–248
    variety and, 241
core exercises, 150–155
crunches, 151–154

dead lift, 136–142
decision fatigue, 58
decline curl-up, 154–155
dehydration, 207–208
diet
    definition of, 199
    focusing on, 21–22
    poor, effects of, 201
    relationship of nutrition, exercise,
        and, 199–200
    See also meal plan
dinner
    considerations for, 231
    examples of, 240, 245, 248
dumbbell exercises
    back extension, 143
    bench press, 120–121
    dead lift, 137, 139–140
    lunge, 146
    row, 125–126
    shoulder press, 127, 128

empty calories, 204
energy
    decision fatigue and, 58
    efficient use of, 21–22
    exercise and, 28
    lack of, 4, 8, 15–16
equipment
    expense of, 40–43
    prepping, 53–54
essential amino acids, 202
essential fatty acids, 206
evaluation concern, 102
evening routine, 61–66
evening workouts, 56–57
exercise
    apprehension about, 37
    benefits of, 27–29, 37, 59–60
    choosing time for, 55–60,
        68–69
    compatible with lifestyle, 27
    daily, 25, 27–29, 33
    equipment, 40–43
    focusing on, 21–22
    frequency of, 25–29
    inadequate, effects of, 201
    mental associations for, 60
    with partners and groups,
        47–48
    proximity of location for, 38–40
    recovery time after, 29, 170, 172
    relationship of nutrition, diet, and,
        199–200
    starting new program of, 116,
        194–195
    supportive tasks for, 37–38
    See also cardio exercise; fitness;
        gyms, home; habits; motivation;
        strength-training exercises;
        workouts

expectations
    muscle development, 95–98
    setting realistic, 89, 104
    weight loss, 93–94
fats
    excess, 206
    muscle development and, 207
    per-meal targets for, 231–233
    recommended daily allowance
        (RDA) for, 207
    role of, 206
    saturated, 206
    sources of, 206, 207, 224
    staples, 223–225
    trans, 206
    unsaturated, 206–207
    See also body fat
FFMI (fat-free mass index)
    adjusted, 81–82
    BMI vs., 80
    calculating, 80–82
    changes in, 106–109, 111
    daily tracking of, 106
    definition of, 80
    muscle development goals and, 89
    muscularity scales for men and
        women, 83
fiber, 204, 205
fitness
    barriers to achieving, 4, 8
    effects of lack of, 13–15
    importance of, 2, 3, 4
    motivation and, 3–5, 11–19
    as ongoing process, 112
    questions about, 14
    short- vs. long-term benefits of,
        17–19
    See also diet; exercise

fitness goals
    importance of, 12
    setting, 73, 84–90
    total goal profiles, 92
    unrealistic, 23
    vague, 11
floor mats, 41–42
free weights, 42
    See also barbell exercises; dumbbell
        exercises
friction
    concept of, 5, 19
    minimizing, 7, 9, 20, 22, 27, 36,
        54
    motivation and, 19–20, 54
    sources of, 37–40, 48–54
    timing and, 55
fruits
    as energy source, 228
    hydration and, 208
    nutrition and, 227

ghrelin, 28
glucose, 204, 205
grains, 227, 228
groups, dependence on, 47–48
gyms, commercial
    advantages of, 40
    cost of memberships at, 40,
        43–44
    nearby, 46–47
    partner/group exercise at,
        47–48
    travel time to, 38–40
gyms, home
    eliminating friction with, 39
    expense of equipment for, 40–43
    hosting group workouts at, 48
    making space for, 44–47
    prepping equipment in, 53–54

habits
    benefits of, 24
    definition of, 24
    frequency and, 25
    friction and, 5
    importance of building sustainable,
        2–3, 5, 23–24, 35, 91, 257–258
    time required to form, 30–33
HDL cholesterol, 206
heart health, 74–75
heart rate
    gauging, 190–192
    manipulating, 192–193
    maximal, 155–156, 190
    monitors, 191
    setting target, 155–156, 189–190
height, measuring, 78
hip-dominant pull, 136–144
hip extensions, 142–143
horizontal pull, 124–127
horizontal push, 120–124
hunger, curbing, 28
hydration, 207–208
hyperextension bench, 142

injury
    changing workout pattern after,
        170
    reducing risk of, 142, 151, 160, 162,
        179, 193
interval training, 156, 186–187,
    188
isolation exercises, 149–150

jumping jacks, 158
jumping rope, 158–159

lactic acid, 75
lateral pull-downs, 131, 132
LDL cholesterol, 206

lean body mass (LBM)
  calculating, 81
  definition of, 81
  protein intake and, 203–204
  target body weight and, 86
Lose It (app), 241
lunch
  considerations for, 231
  examples of, 238, 240, 244, 247
lunch-break workouts, 56
lunges, 145–146

macronutrients
  calculator tool, 210, 211, 213
  caloric content of, 210
  definition of, 93
  per-meal targets for, 231–233
  subcategories of, 202
  See also carbohydrates; fats; protein
meal plan
  building, 235–237, 242
  deviations from, 249–250, 254–256
  examples of, 238–240, 243–248
  meal tracking and, 251–254
  nutrition apps and, 241–242,
    251–254
  per-meal macro targets and,
    231–233
  prep time and, 222–223, 228–229
  simplicity and, 216–217, 241
  traditional approach to, 215–216
  travel and, 255–256
  See also core daily meals; diet;
    nutritional plan; staple foods
meals
  cheat, 249–250
  customary times for, 230–231
  number of per-day, 229–230
  portion sizes and, 252–253
  tracking, 251–254

melatonin, 66
men
  age-based body-fat guidelines for,
    85
  body-fat percentage norms for,
    80
  FFMI muscularity scale for, 83
  "ideal" body type for, 101–102
  measuring body-fat percentage
    for, 79
  recommended protein intake for,
    203
mental capacities, enhancing, 28
MHR (maximal heart rate), 155–156,
  189–191
micronutrients, 209
monounsaturated fats, 206–207
mood, improving, 28
morning workouts, 57–60, 68–69
motivation
  definition of, 35
  establishing lasting, 9, 11–13
  forcing, through willpower,
    35–36
  friction and, 19–20, 54
  identifying sources of, 12,
    15–19
  increasing, 36
  lack of, 11
muscle development
  age and, 98–99
  carbohydrates and, 205
  expectations for, 95–98
  fats and, 207
  myths about, 98–104
  protein and, 203
  setting directional goal for, 87–89,
    92
  strength training and, 76–77, 95,
    174–177, 184–185

muscle mass
  body fat and, 92
  calculating, 80–83
  daily tracking of, 106
  See also FFMI
MyFitnessPal (app), 241

National Weight Control Registry, 27
Neverland fallacy, 98–99
nutrition
  definition of, 199
  inadequate, effects of, 200
  key components of, 201–209
  relationship of diet, exercise, and,
    199–200
  See also carbohydrates; fats;
    protein; vitamins
nutritional plan
  building, 209–211, 213
  examples of, 212
  revising, 211, 213
  See also meal plan
nutrition apps, 241–242, 251–254

obliques, 154

partners, dependence on, 47–48
peptide YY, 28
per-meal macro targets, 231–233
pets, 67
phones, 66
physical fitness. *See* fitness
pike press, 130
polyunsaturated fats, 206–207
portion sizes, 252–253
processed foods, 225
procrastination, overcoming, 59
protein
  composition of, 202
  excess, 203

  muscle development and, 203
  per-meal targets for, 231–233
  prep time and, 222–223
  recommended daily allowance
    (RDA) for, 203–204
  role of, 202
  sources of, 203, 220–221
  staples, 220–223
pull-ups, 131–132, 134–135

quad-dominant push, 145–148

registered dietician (RD), hiring, 219
resistance band exercises
  chin-up, 134
  dead lift, 137, 140–141
  press, 122, 124
  pull-down, 135–136
  row, 125, 126–127
  shoulder press, 127, 129
  squat, 147–148
resistance training. *See* strength-
  training exercises
rest days, 29
Romanian dead lift, 141
room temperature for sleep, 67
rows, 124–127
running in place, 157–158

saturated fats, 206
scales
  as important tool, 78
  measuring body-fat percentage
    with, 79
shoulder press, 127–130
simple carbohydrates, 204
sleep
  environment for, 66–68
  evening routine and, 61–66
  exercise and, 28, 172

lack of, 61
tips for better, 64–66
wakeup time and, 63–64, 68
soreness, 172
squat racks, 43, 122, 131
squats, 145, 147–148
staple foods
benefits of, 217
calorie-efficient, 218–219
carb, 225–229
considerations for, 217–218
definition of, 217
fat, 223–225
prep time and, 222–223, 228–229
protein, 220–223
selecting, 217–219
starches, 204–205, 228
strength-training exercises (anaerobic
exercise)
age and, 98–99, 103–104
benefits of, 76
calibrating resistance for, 177–179
choosing, 117–118, 159–160, 161
compound, 118–120, 150
definition of, 75
determining rep volume for,
174–177
efficient, 118
equipment for, 121–122, 142, 147
examples of, 76
goal for, 77, 89
hip-dominant pull, 136–144
horizontal pull, 124–127
horizontal push, 120–124
increasing resistance for, 183–184
isolation, 149–150
lactic acid and, 75
muscle development and, 76–77,
95, 174–177, 184–185
myths about, 76, 98–104

number of sets for, 173
quad-dominant push, 145–148
resting between sets of, 184–185
splitting, into daily workouts,
172–173
vertical pull, 131–136
vertical push, 127–130
women and, 100, 101–103
stress management, 28
stretching, 194
success, keys to, 3–4, 7–8
sugar, refined, 204
sugar crash, 204
supplements, 209

tea, 208
televisions, 67
time
efficient use of, 21–22
lack of, 4, 8
-saving tips, 62–63
Tracy, Brian, 59
trans fats, 206
travel, 137, 147, 169, 170, 255–256

unsaturated fats, 206

vegetables
green leafy, 228
hydration and, 208
nutrition and, 227
vertical pull, 131–136
vertical push, 127–130
vitamins
carb sources and, 227
deficiencies of, 209
fats and, 206
role of, 209
sources of, 209
supplements, 209

wakeup time, 63–64, 68
warm-ups, 160, 162, 193
water, 207–208
weight bench, 42
weighted lunges, 145–146
weight gain
   nutritional plan and, 211, 213
   weekly goal for, 211
   See also body weight
weightlifting. *See* strength-training
   exercises
weight loss
   burning calories for, 30, 74, 93–94
   calorie deficit and, 93–94
   expectations for, 93–94
   maintaining, 27
   nutritional plan and, 211, 213
   weekly goal for, 211
   See also body weight
whole foods, 225
women
   age-based body-fat guidelines for, 85
   body-fat percentage norms for, 80
   evaluation concern and, 102
   FFMI muscularity scale for, 83
   "ideal" body type for, 101–103
   measuring body-fat percentage for,
      78–79
   recommended protein intake for,
      203
   strength training and, 100, 101–
      103
workouts
   choosing exercises for, 51–52,
      117–118, 159–162
   clothes for, 49–51
   cool-downs after, 193, 194
   daily, 25, 27–29, 33
   documenting performance in,
      53–54, 181–183
   evening, 56–57
   frequency of, 25–29
   group exercises for, 164–169
   heart rate during, 189–193
   incorporating cardio into,
      186–187
   length of, 29–32, 187, 189
   lunch-break, 56
   morning, 57–60, 68–69
   recovery time and, 170, 172
   scheduling, 169–70, 171
   shortening, 31–32
   skipping, 26, 32
   splitting strength-training exercises
      for, 172–173
   warm-ups for, 160, 162, 193

About the Author

TYLER MARTIN is a certified personal trainer and a former high school wrestling coach and collegiate-level athlete. As a coach, he helped young athletes achieve All-State and All-American level accolades and advance to collegiate-level competition.

Tyler's innovative approach to fitness and behavior change enables him to stay in fantastic shape while managing a demanding life as a full-time marketer, business owner, researcher, writer, and husband. His fitness system revolutionized his life by helping him and his family develop lifelong fitness habits that are compatible with busy lifestyles.

After retiring from athletics, Tyler quickly learned that as an average working person, he'd have much less time and energy to devote to maintaining a proper diet and exercise regimen. This realization prompted him to develop a solution for getting and staying in great shape while expending the least amount of effort. He realized the habit-forming methods he learned as an athlete and coach could be applied to basic fitness principles to create a fitness system that is compatible with modern life.

In 2010, Tyler began studying the diet and exercise literature and experimenting with various methods. After many years of being his own guinea pig and identifying what works, he devised an efficient and complete fitness philosophy and system. Soon after, his wife, Morgan, and her family implemented the system, and they all experienced great success. Tyler spent the next five years honing and codifying his approach into a straightforward and comprehensive program for busy people.

Tyler, who lives in Louisville, Kentucky, enjoys laughing with his wife, playing with his dog, Maverick, and having deep discussions with a few good friends. When he has free time, Tyler enjoys reading inspiring novels and watching movies that have great heroes.